The Obstetric Nurse's Survival Guide

Yondell Masten, R.N.C., Ph.D., O.G.N.P.

Brenda Goodner, R.N., M.S.N., C.S.

A SKIDMORE-ROTH PUBLICATION

Publisher: Linda Skidmore-Roth
Cover design: Daniel K. Raffel
Developmental Editor: Alexandra Swann

Notice: The author and publisher of this volume have taken care to make certain that all information is correct and compatible with standards generally accepted at the time of publication. Because the science of nursing is constantly changing and expanding, new techniques and concepts are continually implemented. Therefore, the reader is encouraged to stay abreast of new developments in the nursing field and to be aware that policies vary according to the guidelines of each school or institution.

Goodner, Brenda
The Obstetric Survival Guide

ISBN 0-944132-94-4
1. Nursing Handbooks, Manuals
2. Medical Handbooks, Manuals

SKIDMORE-ROTH PUBLISHING, INC.
7730 Trade Center Ave.
El Paso, Texas 79912
1 (800)825-3150

TABLE OF CONTENTS

INTRODUCTION

ASSESSMENT

CLINICAL SKILLS

TEACHING TOPICS

CLINICAL VALUES AND STANDARDS

DRUG ADMINISTRATION

PROFESSIONAL NETWORK

APPENDIX A: PROFESSIONAL STANDARDS

APPENDIX B: CERVICAL DILATION

INTRODUCTION

INTRODUCTION

HOW TO USE THIS BOOK

The *Obstetric Survival Guide* is a companion to the popular *Nurse's Survival Guide*. This book is not just another spectator manual in nursing written by uninvolved nurses. This is a book that you can really use, especially when confronted with unfamiliar assignments.

This book is about accountability. By having information readily available, it is hoped that the nurse and the nursing student will increase their accountability in situations where they would otherwise feel uncomfortable. Accountability is the hallmark of nursing care, and nurses are constantly being called upon to fulfill the demands that accountability affords.

This book is not intended to replace a nursing textbook. Instead, it will complement textbooks as an easy-to-grab handbook. This book presents information that nurses may use frequently but not necessarily memorize. It is a handbook loaded with guidelines, assessment forms, and charts of information. This book is not intended to offer extensive rationale. When you do not understand the rationale, then is time to research the subject in a comprehensive maternal-child textbook.

THE MARK OF A PROFESSIONAL NURSE

The basic requirements of a profession are:

- ▲ Educational requirements
- ▲ Unique knowledge and skills based upon theory
- ▲ Service to society
- ▲ Autonomy in decision-making and practice
- ▲ A code of ethics for practice
- ▲ Some degree of status within the role

These requirements are inherent in the foundation of professional nursing. The profession of compassionate caring that Florence Nightingale embraced for nursing is the interpersonal expertise unique to each nurse. These interpersonal skills are intimately interwoven with the professional skills. Never are these interpersonal skills more essential than with obstetric nursing.

Interpersonal skills encompass all the human actions that respect the body, mind and spirit of another person. It is looking at the patient with kindness, listening with empathy, and responding with compassion. A professional nurse offers much more than technical skills, although more and more, technical skills are required.

What do patients want in a nurse? This question has been researched, and it has been found that they want empathy, sensitivity, experience (skills), caring and a sense of confidence, in that order. What they do not want is a nurse who is insensitive, in a hurry, with an air of power. Patients tend to feel uncomfortable with nurses who are unsure of what they are doing.

It is impossible to label the characteristic that makes a nurse professional. That essential quality is elusive, perhaps indescribable. But, when you meet a nurse who has it, you know.

STANDARDS OF CLINICAL NURSING PRACTICE

The American Nurses' Association sets a standard for nursing that focuses on practice. When nursing care is measured, accountability is also measured by how these standards are concurrently utilized. The ANA Standards of Clinical Nursing Practice are used for measuring accountability in nursing.

The first standards were published in 1973. In 1989, a task force began revising these standards, and these standards were published in 1991. The major change is the emphasis on clinical nursing practice. The standards now address the full scope of practice and are divided into two parts—Standards of Care and Standards of Professional Performance.

Standards of Care

* Assessment
* Collegiality
* Implementation
* Quality of care
* Education
* Collaboration
* Resource utilization
* Diagnosis
* Planning
* Evaluation
* Performance appraisal
* Ethics
* Research
* Outcome identification

"Standards of Care" describe a competent level of nursing care as demonstrated by the nursing process, involving assessment, nursing diagnosis, outcome identification, planning, implementation, and evaluation. The nursing process encompasses all significant actions taken by nurses in providing care to all clients and forms the foundation of clinical decision-making. Additional nursing responsibilities for all clients (such as providing culturally and ethnically relevant care, maintaining a safe environment, educating clients about their illnesses, treatment, health promotion or self-care activities, and planning for continuity of care) are explained within these standards. Therefore, "Standards of Care" delineate care that is provided to all clients of nursing services.

STANDARDS OF PROFESSIONAL PERFORMANCE

"Standards of Professional Performance" describe a competent level of behavior in the professional role including activities related to quality of care, performance appraisal, education, collegiality, ethics, collaboration, research, and resource utilization. All nurses are expected to engage in professional role activities appropriate to their education, position and practice setting. While this is no assumption of all of the "Standards of Professional Performance", the scope of nursing involvement in some professional roles is particularly dependent upon the nurse's education, position, and practice environment. Therefore, some standards or measurement criteria identify a broad age of activities that may demonstrate compliance with the standards.

STANDARDS OF CARE

STANDARD I. Assessment

The nurse collects client health data.

Measurement Criteria

1. The priority of data collection is determined by the client's immediate condition or needs.
2. Pertinent data are collected using appropriate assessment techniques.
3. Data collection involves the client, significant others, and health care providers, when appropriate.
4. The data collection process is systematic and ongoing.
5. Relevant data are documented in a retrievable form.

STANDARD II. Diagnosis

The nurse analyzes the assessment data in determining diagnoses.

Measurement Criteria

1. Diagnoses are derived from the assessment data.
2. Diagnoses are validated with the client, significant others, and health care providers, when possible.
3. Diagnoses are documented in a manner that facilitates the determination of unexpected outcomes and plan of care.

STANDARD III. Outcome Identification

The nurse identifies expected outcomes individualized to the client.

Measurement Criteria

1. Outcomes are derived from the diagnoses.
2. Outcomes are documented as measurable goals.
3. Outcomes are mutually formulated with the client's present and potential capabilities.
4. Outcomes are realistic in relation to the client's present and potential capabilities.
5. Outcomes are attainable in relation to resources available to the client.
6. Outcomes include a time estimate for attainment.
7. Outcomes provide direction for continuity of care.

STANDARD IV. Planning

The nurse develops a plan of care that prescribes interventions to attain expected outcomes.

Measurement Criteria

1. The plan is individualized to the client's condition or needs.
2. The plan is developed with the client, significant others, and health care providers, when appropriate.
3. The plan reflects current nursing practice.
4. The plan is documented.
5. The plan provides for continuity of care.

STANDARD V. Implementation

The nurse implements the interventions identified in the plan of care.

Measurement Criteria

1. Interventions are consistent with the established plan of care.
2. Interventions are implemented in a safe and appropriate manner.
3. Interventions are documented.

STANDARD VI. Evaluation

The nurse evaluates the client's progress toward attainment of outcomes.

Measurement Criteria

1. Evaluation is systematic and ongoing.
2. The client's responses to interventions are documented.
3. The effectiveness of interventions is evaluated in relation to outcomes.
4. Ongoing assessment data are used to revise diagnoses, outcomes, and the plan of care, as needed.
5. Revisions in diagnoses, outcomes, and the plan of care are documented.
6. The client, significant others, and health care providers are involved in the evaluation process, when appropriate.

STANDARDS OF PROFESSIONAL PERFORMANCE

STANDARD I. Quality of Care

The nurse systematically evaluates the quality and effectiveness of nursing practice.

Measurement Criteria

1. The nurse participates in quality of care activities as appropriate to the individual's position, education, and practice environment. Such activities may include:

   - Identification of aspects of care important for quality monitoring.
   - Identification of indicators used to monitor quality and effectiveness of nursing care.
   - Collection of data to monitor quality and effectiveness of nursing care.
   - Analysis of quality data to identify opportunities for improving care.
   - Formulation of recommendations to improve nursing practice or client outcomes.
   - Implementation of activities to enhance the quality of nursing practice.
   - Participation on interdisciplinary teams that evaluate clinical practice or health services.
   - Development of policies and procedures to improve quality of care.

2. The nurse uses the results of quality of care activities to initiate changes in practice.

3. The nurse uses the results of quality of care activities to initiate changes throughout the health care delivery system, as appropriate.

STANDARD II. Performance Appraisal

The nurse evaluates his/her own nursing practice in relation to professional practice standards and relevant statutes and regulations.

Measurement Criteria

1. The nurse engages in performance appraisal on a regular basis, identifying areas of strength as well as areas for professional/practice development.
2. The nurse seeks constructive feedback regarding his/her own practice.
3. The nurse takes action to achieve goals identified during performance appraisal.
4. The nurse participates in peer review as appropriate.

STANDARD III. Education

The nurse acquires and maintains current knowledge in nursing practice.

Measurement Criteria

1. The nurse participates in ongoing educational activities related to clinical knowledge and professional issues.
2. The nurse seeks experiences to maintain clinical skills.
3. The nurse seeks knowledge and skills appropriate to the practice setting.

STANDARD IV. Collegiality

The nurse contributes to the professional development of peers, colleagues, and others.

Measurement Criteria

1. The nurse shares knowledge and skill with colleagues and others.

2. The nurse provides peers with constructive feedback regarding their practice.

3. The nurse contributes to an environment that is conducive to clinical education of nursing students as appropriate.

STANDARD V. Ethics

The nurse's decisions and actions on behalf of clients are determined in an ethical manner.

Measurement Criteria

1. The nurse's practice is guided by the Code for Nurses.

2. The nurse maintains client confidentiality.

3. The nurse acts as a client advocate.

4. The nurse delivers care in a nonjudgmental and nondiscriminatory manner that is sensitive to client diversity.

5. The nurse delivers care in a manner that preserves/protects client autonomy, dignity, and rights.

6. The nurse seeks available resources to help formulate ethical decisions.

STANDARD VI. Collaboration

The nurse collaborates with the client, significant others and health care providers in providing client care.

Measurement Criteria

1. The nurse communicates with the client, significant others, and health care providers regarding client care and nursing's role in the provision of care.

2. The nurse consults with health care providers for client care, as needed.

3. The nurse makes referrals, including provisions for continuity of care, as needed.

STANDARD VII. Research

The nurse uses research findings in practice.

Measurement Criteria

1. The nurse uses interventions substantiated by research as appropriate to the individual's position, education, and practice environment.

2. The nurse participates in research activities as appropriate to the individual's position, education, and practice environment. Such activities may include:

   - Identification of clinical problems suitable for nursing research

   - Participation in data collection

   - Participation in a unit, organization, or community research committee or program

   - Sharing of research activities with others

   - Conducting research

- Critiquing research for application to practice
- Using research findings in the development of policies, procedures, and guidelines for client care

STANDARD VIII. Resource Utilization

The nurse considers factors related to safety, effectiveness, and cost in planning and delivering client care.

Measurement Criteria

1. The nurse evaluates factors related to safety, effectiveness, and cost when two or more practice options would result in the same expected client outcome.

2. The nurse assigns tasks or delegates care based on the needs of the client and the knowledge and skill of the provider selected.

3. The nurse assists the client and significant others in identifying and securing appropriate services available to address health-related needs.

From the ANA's Standards of Nursing Practice, 1991.

ASSESSMENT

ASSESSMENT

PATIENT HISTORY

Biographical Data

Name _____

Address and phone _____

Social Security number_____

Age, birthdate, birthplace _____

Sex _____

Ethnicity _____

Marital status _____

Significant other/contact person_____

Occupation and education_____

Religion _____

Stability of living conditions _____

Economic status_____

Current Pregnancy History

First day of last menstrual period (LMP) _____

Date, results, and type of pregnancy test _____

Symptoms of pregnancy _____

Bleeding and/or cramping since LMP_____

Vaginal discharge _____

Personal risk factors _____

Environmental risk factors _____

Maternal health risk factors _____

Maternal current/past gestational risk factors _____

_____

Maternal feelings regarding pregnancy _____

First day of last normal menstrual period (LNMP), if LMP were not normal in terms of length of menstrual cycle, amount of bleeding, and/or duration of menses_____

Past Pregnancy History

Number of pregnancies_____

Number of term deliveries _____

Number of preterm deliveries _____

Number of abortions (induced, spontaneous) _____

Number of living children _____

For Each Pregnancy

Date of delivery_____

Gestational duration _____

Gestational complications_____

Length and type (induced, augmented, spontaneous) of labor _____

Type of delivery _____

Type of anesthesia_____

Birthweight and gestational age_____

Prenatal, intrapartal, postpartal, neonatal complications ___

_____

Type of complications _____

Current health of child _____

Gynecologic History

Age of menarche _____

Length of menstrual cycle _____

Duration and amount of menses _____

History of dysmenorrhea _____

Previous surgery _____

Previous infection _____

Contraceptive history _____

Date of last Pap smear and results _____

Sexual History

Age at first intercourse _____

Number and health status of sexual partners _____

Number and health status of partner's partners _____

Satisfaction with intercourse _____

Dyspareunia _____

Current Medical History

General health status_____

Nutritional status _____

Exercise habits_____

Health promotion habits _____

Use of tobacco, alcohol, street drugs _____

Use of over-the-counter drugs _____

Current prescribed medications _____

Drug and other allergies _____

Disease conditions_____

Past Medical History

Surgeries_____

Injuries _____

Major illnesses_____

Childhood diseases _____

Immunizations _____

Disease conditions_____

Blood transfusions_____

Developmental History

Cognitive level_____

Psychological status _____

Interpersonal relationships _____

Coping strategies_____

Personal stressors_____

Nutritional history _____

24-hour diet recall_____

Nutritional problems _____

Family Medical History

Multiple births_____

Cesarean births _____

Three generation family genogram:

Congenital diseases _____

Congenital anomalies _____

Disease conditions_____

Cause and age of deaths_____

Current health status of living members_____

Occupational History

Exposure to teratogenic substances _____

_____

Type of work_____

Frequency and duration of rest periods_____

Meal breaks _____

Partner's Current and Past Medical History

Age _____

Ethnicity_____

Occupation _____

Educational level _____

Blood type and Rh factor_____

Disease conditions_____

Use of tobacco, alcohol, street drugs _____

Genetic conditions_____

Perception of the pregnancy_____

Partner's Family Medical History

Disease conditions_____

Congenital diseases _____

Congenital anomalies _____

Genetic disorders_____

Social and Cultural History

Language spoken _____

Support system _____

Housing _____

Living environment _____

Maternal attitude toward pregnancy _____

Extended family/support system attitude toward pregnancy

_____

Religiously-based health beliefs _____

Religiously-based pregnancy health beliefs _____

Culturally-based health beliefs _____

_____

Culturally-based pregnancy health beliefs _____

_____

Knowledge regarding pregnancy and parenting _____

_____

Biographical Information

Name _____

Address and phone _____

Social Security number _____

Age, birthdate, birthplace _____

Sex _____

Ethnicity _____

Marital status _____

Significant other/contact person _____

Occupation and education _____

Religion _____

Stability of living conditions _____

Economic status_____

Chief Complaint

Symptoms of gestational complication _____

Symptoms of labor _____

Frequency and duration of contractions _____

Location of discomfort _____

Quality of fetal movement _____

Status of amniotic membranes _____

Presence and character of vaginal discharge _____

Pregnancy History

First day of last menstrual period (LMP) _____

Date, results, and type of pregnancy test _____

Symptoms of pregnancy _____

Bleeding and/or cramping since LMP_____

Vaginal discharge _____

Personal risk factors _____

Environmental risk factors _____

Maternal health risk factors _____

Maternal current/past gestational risk factors_____

_____

Maternal feelings regarding pregnancy _____

_____

First day of last normal menstrual period (LNMP), if LMP were not normal in terms of length of menstrual cycle, amount of bleeding, and/or duration of menses_____

Prenatal Care History

Gestational age at initiation of prenatal care _____

_____

Frequency of prenatal visits_____
Gestational complications, treatments and outcome_____

_____

Past Medical History

Surgeries_____
Injuries _____
Major illnesses_____
Childhood diseases _____
Immunizations _____
Disease conditions_____
Blood transfusions_____

ADMISSION PATIENT HISTORY

The admission patient history needs to be taken only once and is useful when making referrals. The background information gathered will be helpful when performing the physical assessment.

Biographical

Name _____

Age _____

Sex _____

Nationality _____

Significant other _____

Religion _____

Social Security number_____

Occupation _____

Marital status _____

Referred by _____

Reliability of informant _____

Doctor's name, address_____

Chief Complaint

What specific problem caused you to seek help today?

How long has this been a problem?

(Record as a quote exactly what the patient says)

_____

_____

_____

_____

Detailed History of Illness

What: What were you doing at the time the problem occurred?

When: When did it begin (date, time of day)?

How: Was it a recurring or sudden onset? Severity?

Why: Any precipitating events that occurred?

Past Health History

Major illness (diabetes, cardiac) _____

Injuries in the past_____

Hospitalizations _____

Surgeries_____

Allergies_____

Immunizations _____

Habits: Caffeine, alcohol, drugs, cigarettes_____

Present medications (including over-the-counter) _____

Nutrition _____

Diet _____

Weight loss or gain_____

Significant family illness/death _____

Psychological History

Ability to understand _____

Ability to learn _____

Ability to remember _____

Coping mechanisms _____

Response to illness _____

Past coping patterns _____

Abusive/preventive lifestyle _____

Sociological History

Significant relationships _____

Persons living at home _____

Recent crises/changes at home or work _____

Work environment: Stress/Satisfaction _____

Economic status_____

Adequate financial resources _____

Perception of financial needs _____

Financial strain of illness _____

Cultural/religious implications _____

Food preparation _____

Special rituals _____

Special religious days _____

PSYCHOSOCIAL HISTORY

Household Information

People living in home_____

Length of time at present residence _____

Individual who is emotionally supportive_____

Relationships at home_____

Major stressors at home _____

_____

Number of times each partner has been married _____

Number of children of each partner _____

Cultural Background

Place of birth_____

If foreign country, time in USA and cultural practices
that should be honored _____

Religious preference and background including rituals
that should be honored (such as fasting) _____

_____

Educational Background

Highest degree of each parent _____

Plans for continued education _____

Occupations of Persons Living in The Household

Number of hours worked per week, shift work, hours
involved _____

HISTORY OF HEALTH HABITS

Food and Nutrition

Height, Weight

Ideal weight _____

Recent loss or gain in weight _____

Dieting _____

History of eating disorder_____

Fluid intake/day, including kinds of fluids _____

Snack foods _____

History of fasting _____

Vitamins: Kind, amount, reason for taking_____

Sleep

Hours per night _____

Insomnia_____

Exercise

Kind _____

Amount_____

Frequency_____

Environmental Hazards

Physical _____

Chemical _____

Biological _____

Smoking

Packs/day _____

Kind or brand of cigarettes _____

Age started _____

Attempts to quit: Number/method _____

Number of other smokers at home _____

Are you thinking of stopping now?_____

Alcohol

What kind of alcohol (liquor, beer, wine)? _____

When do you drink? _____

How much do you drink?_____

Do you drink to feel good? _____

How old were you when you started drinking?_____

Do you drink with others or alone? _____

How old were you the first time you got drunk? ____

Have you ever had a problem with drinking? _____

Do you think you have a problem with drinking?_____

Does your partner, or other family members, drink?_____

Have you ever been arrested when drinking? _____

Has anyone ever criticized you for drinking? _____

Have you ever needed a drink in the morning?_____

Drug Use

Do you use drugs for recreational purposes? _____

What kind of drugs do you use? _____

Has doing drugs ever caused you a problem? _____

How old were you when you started using? _____

Do you use marijuana? Cocaine? Heroine? _____

If so, how are these drugs used? _____

Do you shoot IV drugs? _____

How much are you using a week? _____

When do you use drugs? _____

Have you ever smoked crack? _____

Have you ever shared needles? _____

How much are you doing? _____

How much do drugs cost you per week? _____

Over-The-Counter Drugs

Names_____

Frequency of use _____

Reason for taking medication_____

ANTEPARTAL ASSESSMENT

This assessment should be performed during each patient visit.

Physical exam

Blood pressure_____

Urine_____

Weight gain _____

Output _____

Edema _____

Bacteria _____

TPR_____

Protein _____

Fetal heart rate_____

Specific gravity _____

Are you experiencing:

- Headaches
- Nausea/vomiting
- Blurred vision
- Diarrhea
- Leg cramping
- Back pain
- Vaginal bleeding
- Genital ulcerations
- Exposure to infections

- Dizziness
- Heartburn
- Constipation
- Abdominal cramping
- Contractions
- Problems urinating
- Vaginal discharge
- Genital rash, itching
- Fetal movement

Do you have any concerns regarding:

Sexual activity _____

Fetal movement _____

Weight gain _____

Nutritional status _____

Estimated date of delivery (EDD)

Are you taking any:

Prescribed medications _____

Over-the-counter medications _____

Laxatives or enemas _____

Nutritional supplements _____

Vitamins and minerals _____

Alcohol beverages _____

Illicit drugs _____

Are you smoking cigarettes? _____

How are you feeling emotionally:

Support system _____

Abusive behavior _____

Getting enough rest _____

Schedule for Antepartal Care

Appointment	Nulliparas (in weeks)	Multiparas (in weeks)
First	6-8	6-8
Second	12	14-16
Third	14-16	24-28
Fourth	24-28	32
Fifth	32	36
Sixth	36	39
Seventh	38	41
Eighth	40	
Ninth	41	

Schedule will vary for high-risk pregnancies

PSYCHOLOGICAL HISTORY

How do you feel about being pregnant?_____

Is the father emotionally supportive of you? _____

How are you doing emotionally?_____

Have you ever been depressed?_____

Are you feeling depressed now? _____

How would you rate your quality of life at present on a scale of 1-10? _____

If less than 10, what would it take to make it a 10? What do you wish were different?_____

Have you had any major losses in the last 3 years—jobs, family, friends, moving, abortions, miscarriages? _____

_____

Have you ever been in therapy? _____

Have you sustained any significant losses in your life? ___

_____

History of Abuse

Is your partner abusive? _____

Have you been hit or knocked down at any time during your pregnancy? _____

If your partner is abusive, how is this abuse exhibited?___

_____

Are you afraid of your partner?_____

Do you think your partner is in control of you and the relationship?_____

Who controls the money?_____

Have you ever been raped? _____

Do you have any abnormal fears or phobias? _____

_____

Have you ever suffered emotional trauma related to elective or spontaneous abortion?_____

THE INITIAL INTERVIEW

The purpose of the patient interview initially is to gather data, establish rapport and lay a foundation for trust between the patient and the nurse. An expression of warmth and respect by the nurse facilitates this exchange. The nurse must clearly state any expectations and assess the patient's understanding of the communication.

Give the person special attention at the beginning of the interview by calling the patient by name and using appropriate touch.

- Provide for privacy.
- Do not ask one question after another.
- Encourage the patient to talk by using silence.
- A nonjudgmental attitude is essential.
- Avoid long interviews; the patient may get tired or bored.
- Ask only one question at a time to avoid confusion.
- Avoid leading questions that suggest an expected answer.
- Avoid yes or no questions; open-ended ones are usually best.
- Use positive nonverbal communication, such as leaning forward and talking at the same eye level or maintaining eye contact without staring.
- Smile, use light humor when appropriate.

- Do not state opinions or give advice.
- Tell the patient how this information will be used.
- Actively listen to what the patient says and how she says it.
- Be aware of anxiety exhibited as nervous laughing and restlessness.
- Clarify statements when necessary, but avoid confrontation.
- Repeat important points you want the patient to remember.
- Reward the patient with positive comments at the end of the interview.

SCHEDULED PRENATAL ASSESSMENTS

First trimester

Prepregnancy weight _____

Weight gain _____

Blood pressure _____

Urine screen _____

Date of fetal heart rate detection with doppler _____

Minor discomforts _____

Psychosocial responses _____

Danger signs _____

Maternal serum alpha-fetoprotein screen _____

CBC, Type and Rh _____

Rubella titer _____

General antibody screen _____

Urine culture and sensitivity _____

Pap smear _____

Coomb's for Rh negative mother _____

Sickle cell screen for Black mother _____

Second Trimester (Every 4 weeks for low risk)

Weight gain _____

Blood pressure _____

Fetal heart rate (FHR) _____

Date of first FHR detection with fetoscope _____

Urine screen _____

Fundal height _____

Quickening date _____

Fetal movements _____

Minor discomforts _____

Psychosocial responses _____

Danger signs _____

Third Trimester (every 4 weeks to 32 weeks; every 2 weeks from 32-36 weeks; weekly from 36 weeks to birth for low risk)

Weight gain _____

Blood pressure _____

FHR _____

Fetal movements _____

Fetal presentation (32 weeks to birth)_____

Fundal height _____

Blood glucose screen (latter second trimester or early third 24-28 weeks) _____

Hgb and hmt at 28 weeks _____

Coomb's for Rh negative mother _____

Minor discomforts _____

Psychosocial responses _____

Danger signs _____

ASSESSMENT RELATED TO
GENETIC COUNSELING

Family history of a genetic disorder _____

Fetal anomalies detected by ultrasound _____

Pregnancy at age 35 or older _____

Abnormal maternal serum alpha-fetoprotein screen_____

Birth defects in other children: single anomalies, multiple
defect patterns _____

History of metabolic disorders in family _____

Mental retardation or developmental delay in any other
children in family _____

Chronic neurologic or neuromuscular childhood disorder__
_____

Short stature or dysmorphic features_____
_____

Ambiguous genitalia or abnormal sexual development_____
_____

Carrier status for a genetic disease in specific populations
_____

Infertility, sterility, multiple pregnancy losses, or stillbirth
_____

Exposure to potentially mutagenic or teratogenic agents __
_____

Genetic risk due to consanguinity _____

Adult-onset disability of genetic origin_____

Behavioral disorders of genetic origin _____

Cancer, heart disease, and other common conditions with
a genetic component _____

NUTRITIONAL ASSESSMENT

Diet dramatically affects a person's state of health. To assess a patient's nutritional status, first record the typical 24-hour intake, then assess eating habits on a weekly basis. After completing the assessment, you can evaluate the adequacy of the diet according to the guidelines established by the basic food groups.

Nutrition for the pregnant woman consists of eating a well-balanced diet based on the basic food groups. Specific needs for pregnancy and lactation are noted in additional requirements listed in the RDA.

Name _____

Age/Sex _____

Marital status _____

Occupation _____

Height and weight _____

Recent weight loss _____

Medical diagnosis _____

Food restrictions (medical or religious) _____

Ethnic and economic background _____

Problems with eating, general conditions of teeth _____

Food allergies _____

Food preferences _____

Daily nutritional supplements_____

Patient complaints (weakness, indigestion, skin problems)

_____

Elimination habits _____

Use of laxatives_____

Pregnancy Weight Gain

The graph plots weight gain by prenatal visit with the pounds of weight gain on the vertical left axis from -5 or -10 up to 40 or 50 pounds with zero being the prepregnancy weight; the horizontal axis is 0 to 43 weeks gestation.

Recommended weight gain is based on body mass index (BMI) with 1-3 pounds weight gain in the first trimester and the remainder for the second and third trimesters based on the BMI (Institute of Medicine, 1990):

Low BMI (> 19.8) = 28-40 lbs (1-1.5 lbs/wk)

Normal BMI (19.8 - 26.0) = 25-35 lbs (0.9-1.3 lbs/wk)

High BMI (26.0 - 29.0) = 15.25 lbs (0.5-0.9 lbs/wk)

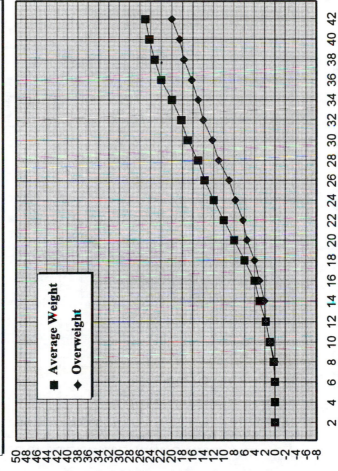

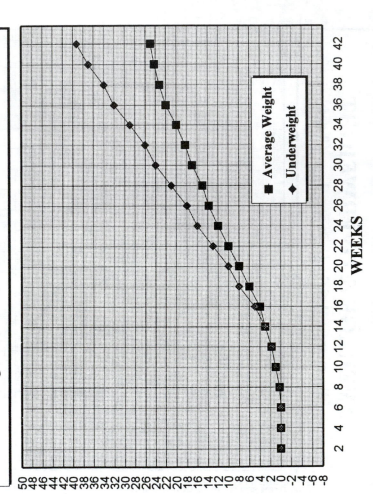

AVERAGE & UNDERWEIGHT
Pregnancy Weight Gain and Loss Chart

HEIGHT AND WEIGHT CHART

Metropolitan Life
Insurance Company

In 1983 the Metropolitan Life Insurance Company devised a height-weight scale that has become a standard.

WOMEN

HEIGHT		FRAME		
Ft.	In.	Small	Medium	Large
4	10	102-111	109-121	118-131
4	11	103-113	111-123	120-134
5	0	104-115	113-126	122-137
5	1	106-118	115-129	125-140
5	2	108-121	118-132	128-143
5	3	111-124	121-135	131-147
5	4	114-127	124-138	134-151
5	5	117-130	127-141	137-155
5	6	120-133	130-144	140-159
5	7	123-136	133-147	143-163
5	8	126-139	136-150	146-167
5	9	129-142	139-153	149-170
5	10	132-145	142-156	152-173
5	11	135-148	145-159	155-176
6	0	138-151	148-162	158-179

MEN

HEIGHT		FRAME		
Ft.	In.	Small	Medium	Large
5	2	128-134	131-141	138-150
5	3	130-136	133-143	140-153
5	4	132-138	135-145	142-156
5	5	134-140	137-148	144-160
5	6	136-142	139-151	146-164
5	7	138-145	142-145	149-168
5	8	140-148	145-157	152-172
5	9	142-151	148-160	155-176
5	10	144-154	151-163	158-180
5	11	146-157	154-166	161-184
6	0	149-160	157-170	164-188
6	1	152-164	160-174	168-192
6	2	155-168	164-178	172-197
6	3	158-172	167-182	176-202
6	4	162-176	171-187	181-207

BISHOP'S SCALE

Bishop's scale for assessing women for induction of labor:

Score	0	1	2	3
Dilatation (cm)	0	1-2	3-4	5-6
Effacement (%)	0-30	40-50	60-70	80
Station (cm)	-3	-2	-1	+1
Cervical consistency	Firm	Medium	Soft	
Fetal position	Posterior	Midline	Anterior	

**Parous woman can be induced at score of 5; nulliparous woman at score of 7.

ASSESSING COMPLICATIONS OF PREGNANCY

- Bleeding anytime, but especially after 20 weeks
- Nutrition
- Hydramnios
- Hypertension
- Rh-negative mother
- Vital infections
- Bacterial infections
- Postmaturity
- Anemia

- Premature rupture of membranes
- No prenatal care
- Excessive weight loss
- Hyperglycemia
- Exposure to teratogens
- Syphilis
- HIV infected
- Abnormal presentation

PRENATAL RISK FACTORS

There are certain factors that are associated with increased morbidity and mortality of mothers and infants. These factors should be carefully monitored if assessed during the initial interviews:

Maternal Characteristics:

- Age: under 18 or over 35
- Ambivalence toward pregnancy
- Low socio-economic group
- Not married
- Family conflict
- 20% overweight or underweight: inadequate nutrition

Obstetric History

- More than one abortion
- Stillbirth
- Infant less than 2500 g
- Infant with major disease
- Preeclampsia or eclampsia
- Difficult deliveries

- Gravidity over 8
- Neonatal death
- Infant over 4,000 g
- Antepartal
- Genital tract anomaly
- Ovarian masses

Medical problems

- Hypertension: Renal
- Heart disease
- Anemia
- Disease: Diabetes mellitus

- Endocrine disorder
- Sickle cell disease
- Pulmonary disease

CLINICAL SKILLS

CLINICAL SKILLS

LEOPOLD'S MANEUVERS

Leopold's maneuvers are four maneuvers implemented to assess fetal position by manually palpating the abdomen. This assessment is used to identify fetal presentation, lie, presenting part, attitude, degree of descent, an estimate of the size, and number of fetuses.

- ❖ Determine lie: longitudinal or transverse
- ❖ Determine location of the head, back, buttocks
- ❖ Determine the presenting part
- ❖ Determine engagement of the presenting part
- ❖ Size of fetus compared to gestational age
- ❖ Determine if more than one fetus is present
- ❖ Determine PMI for fetus
- ❖ Auscultate FHR
- ❖ Determine if fundal height is congruent with gestational age

First maneuver

- ❖ Patient in supine position with knees slightly flexed
- ❖ Put towel under head and right hip
- ❖ With both hands, palpate upper abdomen and fundus
- ❖ Assess size, shape, movement and firmness of the part
- ❖ Head is firm and moveable, breech is soft, less mobile

Second maneuver

❖ With both hands moving down, identify the back

❖ Note whether back is on left or right side of abdomen

Third maneuver

❖ With the right hand over the symphysis pubis, identify the presenting part by grasping the lower abdomen with thumb and fingers

❖ Assess whether the presenting part is engaged in the pelvis (if the head is engaged it will not be moveable)

Fourth maneuver

❖ The nurse alters position by turning toward the patient's feet

❖ With both hands, assess the descent of the presenting part by locating the cephalic prominence or brow

❖ When the brow is on the same side as the back, the head is extended. When the brow is on the same side as the small parts, the head will be flexed and the vertex presenting

TIPS FOR PERFORMING MANEUVERS

❖ Tell the patient where the fetal heartbeat is found and allow her to listen

❖ Tell the patient what is assessed: where the head, the back and buttocks are located.

❖ Instruct to void before procedure to prevent discomfort.

Apgar Scoring System			
	0	**1**	**2**
Heart Rate	Absent	Slow (less than 100 beats/min.)	Greater than 100 beats/min.
Respiratory Effort	Absent	Slow or Irregular	Good: Crying Lustily
Muscle Tone	Limp	Some Flexion of Extremities	Active Motion: Well flexed
Reflex Irritability	No Response	Grimace	(Cough or sneeze) vigorous cry
Color	Blue or pale	Body pink, Extremities Blue	Completely Pink

Breathing Techniques

Breathing techniques are used for relaxation in the early phases of labor. As labor progresses, breathing increases abdominal pressure and aids in the delivery of the fetus.

Dilatation to 3 cm:

- Take cleansing breath (breathe in through the nose and out through the mouth with lips pursed.)
- Keep breathing slow and rhythmic, about 8-10 breaths per minute during each contraction.
- When the contraction ends, take one deep breath and then breathe normally.

Dilatation 4-7 cm:

- Take cleansing breath at the beginning of each contraction
- Breathing becomes more shallow with a rate of about 16 per minute. (Caution against hyperventilation.)
- Encourage slow, abdominal breathing, especially in between contractions.

Dilatation of 8-10 cm:

- Always start with a cleansing breath.
- Maintain concentration or breathing as contractions intensify
- Encourage use of 4:1 breathing pattern: breath, breath, breath, and puff.
- Panting breaths are encouraged to keep mother from pushing down before full dilation is achieved.

DANGER SIGNS DURING LABOR

The labor and delivery nurse should be alert for any deviation from normal. The most common danger signs are:

- ❖ Intrauterine pressure above 75 mm Hg
- ❖ Contractions occuring more than every 2 minutes before transition phase
- ❖ Contractions lasting longer than 60 seconds
- ❖ Fetal bradycardia or tachycardia
- ❖ Irregular fetal heart rate
- ❖ Absence of fetal heartbeat
- ❖ Bloody or greenish amniotic fluid
- ❖ Prolapsed umbilical cord
- ❖ Stop in the descent of the fetus
- ❖ Lack of progress in dilatation and/or effacement

FUNDAL HEIGHT MEASUREMENT

- ❖ Use nonstretchable tape measure.
- ❖ Measure from notch of symphysis pubis to top of the fundus.
- ❖ Be careful not to tip back the corpus.
- ❖ To determine duration of pregnancy in weeks, use McDonald's rule (during the second and third trimester): Height of fundus in cm $\times$ $8/7$ = weeks of pregnancy.

UMBILICAL CORD CARE

❖ Wipe stump area with alcohol-soaked cotton ball every day to promote drying.

❖ Let area air dry.

❖ Fold diaper down to prevent contact with stump area.

❖ Observe for signs and symptoms of infection.

❖ Do not give tub bath until stump falls off.

❖ Stump usually falls off in 10 days.

❖ Do not, under any circumstances, attempt to forcefully remove the cord.

CARDIOPULMONARY RESUSCITATION
ONE RESCUER CPR, ADULT

ASSESSMENT	ACTION
1. **Airway.** Determine Unresponsiveness Call for help Position victim Open airway	Shake shoulder, *"Are you ok?"* Call out, **"Help!"** Turn to supine position. Use head-tilt/chin-lift maneuver.

2. **Breathing**
    Determine:
    Breathlessness
    Ventilate

    Ear over mouth, observe
    chest: Look, listen. Feel for
    breathing *(3-5 seconds.)* Seal
    mouth and nose. Ventilate 2
    times at a rate of 1-1.5
    seconds per inspiration.
    Watch chest rise for adequate
    ventilation.

3. **Circulation**
    Determine:
    Pulselessness
    Activate EMS
    Begin chest
    Compressions.

    Check carotid 5-10 seconds.
    Maintain head tilt. If
    someone has responded, send
    them for help. Check
    landmark for hand placement
    two fingers above xyphoid
    process. Compress 1 1/2-2".
    Compression rate: 80-100
    min. *(Same procedure as one
    man.)*

4. **Compression:**
    Ventilation Ratio

    15-2. 15 compressions and 2
    ventilations. Do 4 cycles and
    check carotid (5 seconds.) If
    no pulse, continue CPR.

TWO RESCUER CPR; ADULT

ASSESSMENT	ACTION
1. Airway *(Same procedure as one man)*	
2. Breathing *(Same procedure as one man.)*	
3. Circulation Determine Pulselessness. Compressor gets into position.	Say "No pulse."Check landmark.
4. Compression/ Ventilation Ratio	Ratio: 5-1. Rate: 80-100/min. Say any mnemonic. Stop compression to allow for each ventilation. Ventilator ventilates after every 5 compressions. After 10 cycles, ventilator checks carotid pulse.
5. Call for switch	Compressor calls for switch. compressor completes 5th compression. Ventilator completes ventilation, then switches.

| 6. | **Switch** | Ventilator moves to chest and compressor moves to head in simultaneous movement. New ventilator checks carotid. Say, "NO pulse" ventilate once. Continue CPR. |

ONE RESCUER CPR, INFANT

ASSESSMENT	ACTION
1. Airway *(Same procedure as one man adult)*	Be careful not to hyperextend the head. Ventilate twice.
2. Breathing *(Same procedure as one man adult)*	**EXCEPTION:** Make tight seal around nose and mouth.
3. Circulation Determine Pulselessness. Activate EMS Begin chest Compression.	Feel for brachial pulse for 5-10 seconds. Draw imaginary line between nipples. Place 2-3 fingers on sternum, 1 finger's width below imaginary line. Compress vertically, 1/2-1". Say any helpful mnemonic. Compression rate: 100/min

4. **Compression/
    Ventilation Ratio**

Ratio: 5-1. 5 compressions
to 1 slow ventilation.
Pause for ventilation Do
ten cycles, then check
brachial pulse. No pulse:
Ventilate once. Continue
CPR

FETAL MONITORING

Stage	FHT range/method	FHT Changes/Cause	Interventions
Antepartum	120-160 bpm heard at 12 weeks with doppler, at 20 weeks with fetoscope		Monitored at prenatal visits
Intrapartum **Stage I Labor Latent Phase**	120-160 bpm with fetoscope, external fetal monitor	Variability in rate during fetal movement and uterine contractions. Baseline of 120 bpm (bradycardia), 160 bpm (tachycardia)	Heard below umbilicus taken by fetoscope to identify baseline. Requires continuous electronic fetal monitoring and action for late deceleration

Stage 1 Labor Active Transition Phases	120-160 bpm with fetoscope, external fetal monitor	Some rate variations in response to fetal movement and contractions; some late deceleration or acceleration with electronic fetal monitoring	Heard below umbilicus or symphysis pubis based on fetal descent
Early in stage	As low as 110 bpm by electronic fetal monitoring (deceleration)	Early deceleration caused by prolonged fetal head compression if descent is 1 cm/hr primigravida 2 cm/hr multigravida	Assess tracing for onset early in contraction, return to baseline by end of contraction. Compare tracing with FHT by doptone, contractions by palpation

Stage II Labor Expulsion of Fetus	Rate based on fetal hypoxia (declaration) by fetal monitoring	Late deceleration caused by impaired uterine circulation	Assess tracing for slowing 20-30 seconds after start of contraction and return to baseline by end of contraction
	Rate based on cord compression (variable)	Variable deceleration with slowing or speeding up caused by degree or severity of contractions	O_2/face mask at 4L/min, consent signed for internal monitoring, position in left-side lying or knee-chest, remain with patient

	Repeated late declaration or variable declaration	Prolonged variable deceleration or late declaration (100 bpm), reduced variability of 5 bpm caused by cord compression, indicates fetal hypoxia	Notify physician, prepare for forcep delivery if completely dilated, absence of prolapsed cord, membranes ruptured, or prepare for C-section
Stage II Labor Expulsion of fetus	120-160 bpm by fetoscope, continuous external monitor	May vary 6-10 bpm during birth with bradycardia during contractions, with return to baseline after contraction Rate after birth 100 bpm unless infant is compromised by uterine/ placental insufficiency	Perform APGAR scoring 1 and 5 minutes after birth

ESTIMATED DATE OF DELIVERY

Nägele's rule uses the first day of the last menstrual period (LMP) or the first day of the last normal menstrual period (LNMP) if the last menstrual period were abnormal in terms of amount or duration of menses. The EDD determined by Nägele's Rule adds 7 days to the first day of the LMP, subtracts 3 months from the month of the LMP and adds 1 year to the year of the LMP. The calculated EDD is then considered correct within 2 weeks. An example would be a client with the first day of her LMP being July 4, 1994. The calculation would be the following:

	Month	Day	Year
LMP	7	4	1994
EDD	-3	+7	+1
	4	11	1995

Thus, the EDD would be April 11, 1995, and birth could be expected within 2 weeks before or 2 weeks after April 11. If the uterine size is approximately the same as the calculated weeks of gestation, then the data indicate uterine size and EDD date consistency (abbreviated as size-date consistency or S=D)

STAGES OF LABOR AND ASSOCIATED CHANGES

STAGE I (LATENT PHASE)	CHANGES 8 1/2 h
Mild, better coordinated contractions (manually or electronically monitored)	Contractions 5-30 min apart, lasting 10-30 sec
Cervical dilatation and effacement Fern test of vaginal secretions (sterile vaginal exam unless bleeding or ruptured membranes present)	Dilatation 0-3 cm, complete effacement in primigravida, effacement with dilatation in multigravida, yellow-to-blue color change
Station (measured above or below ischial spines)	Nitrazine paper (positive Fern test) and rupture of membranes
Mucus plug	Degree of descent 0-2 cm with primigravida experiencing slower rate with little or no descent Pinkish or brownish mucus with increased secretions
Ruptured or intact membranes	May have ruptured before this time

STAGES OF LABOR AND ASSOCIATED CHANGES

Position and presentation of fetus (performing Leopold's maneuver)	Position may be occiput left or right, anterior or posterior (OLA, ORA, OLP, ORP), sacrum right posterior (SRO), or other; presentation may be vertex, breech, shoulder
Fetal heart tones	Between 120-160 bpm heard at umbilicus or slightly lower with increases during fetal movement and uterine contractions
Pulse and blood pressure	Remains at baseline levels
Stage I Labor (Active Phase)	**Changes 5-6 h primigravida, as little as 2 h multigravida**
Moderate, regular fundal dominant contractions	Contractions 2-3 min apart, lasting 45-60 seconds
Cervical dilatation, Friedman graph (rectal exam)	Dilatation 4-8 cm, usually 1-2 cm/hr in primigravida, 1.5 cm/hr in multigravida, Friedman graph used to correlate dilatation with fetal descent

STAGES OF LABOR AND ASSOCIATED CHANGES

Station (below ischial spines)	Descent into midpelvis 0-2, at least 1 cm/hr in primigravida, 2 cm/hr in multigravida
Vaginal secretions	Moderate to large amounts of bloody mucus, some amniotic fluid if membranes have ruptured
Fetal heart tones between contractions	Between 120-160 bpm heard just below umbilicus depending on fetal position with rate responding to contractions and fetal movement.
Vital Signs	Usually at baseline levels but hypotension may occur as a result of regional block
Stage I Labor (Transition Phase)	**Changes 2 hour in primigravida; 1 hour in multigravida**
Strong and lasting contractions	Contractions 3-5 min apart, lasting 30-45 sec
Cervical dilatation, urge to push	Dilatation 8-10 cm, with pushing discouraged until cervix is completely dilated

STAGES OF LABOR AND ASSOCIATED CHANGES

Station and effacement	Station of 2 to 3 with descent of 2-3 cm as percentage of effacement increases
Vaginal secretions	Large amounts bloody mucus
Fetal heart tones between or after each contraction	Between 120-160 bpm heard slightly above symphysis pubis, rate changes if uterine circulation impaired (decelerated late in the state) or if fetal head is compressed (decelerated early in the stage)
Vital signs in between contractions	Slight elevation in pulse and respirations with panting, increased bpm of 10 mm Hg over baseline

STAGES OF LABOR AND ASSOCIATED CHANGES

Stage II Labor (Expulsion of Fetus)	Changes 1 hour in primigravida; 15 minutes in multigravida
Strong, extremely uncomfortable contractions	Contractions 2-3 minutes apart, lasting 60-90 seconds
Cervical dilatation and effacement	Dilatation 10 cm with complete effacement
Station and fetal position	Station reaching 4 as head reaches perineal floor
Vaginal secretions	Copious bloody mucus and increased amniotic fluid expelled during contractions
Crowning with urge to push	Perineal bulging, flattening as fetus descends with head visible
Fetal heart tones after each contraction	Between 120-160 bpm with variations of 6-10 bpm, bradycardia may occur during contractions
Vital signs between contractions	Increased 5-10 mm Hg systolic increase in BP

STAGES OF LABOR AND ASSOCIATED CHANGES

Birth of infant, position and presentation	Episiotomy may be done to facilitate birth, prevent tearing; forceps may be used if stage is prolonged or pushing is inhibited; baby's body will rotate following expulsion of the head, and rest of body is expelled; cord is cut and infant is evaluated by APGAR and placed in warm bassinet
Stage III (Expulsion of placenta)	**Changes 2-3 minutes after birth or after 1st or 2nd contraction as placenta separation takes place**
Contractions, height and shape of uterus	Fundus of uterus rises in the abdomen, changes to globular shape

STAGES OF LABOR AND ASSOCIATED CHANGES

Umbilical cord, uterine bleeding	Cord protrudes and lengthens, blood may trickle or gush from behind, separating placenta with a loss of 250-300 mnts separation from inner to outer margins, or Duncan mechanism presents separation from outer margins, inward
Mechanism of placental expulsion, intactness, abnormalities	Increases in response to changes in cardiac output, which increases 30% during labor, decreases 15-25% after birth, BP and P return to normal after placental expulsion is completed
Stage IV (Immediate postpartum)	**Changes 1-2 hours after delivery**
Uterine height, tone position	Uterine fundus at umbilicus, positioned in midline; firm, contracted, or becomes firm when massaged
Lochia	Moderate amount of rubra; vaginal bleeding with occasional clots

STAGES OF LABOR AND ASSOCIATED CHANGES	
Perineum	Episiotomy or laceration present; some soreness, edema, ecchymosis possible
Bladder distention	Fullness may displace fundus upward and cause boggy or relaxed uterus
Breasts	Soft with erect nipples, breast feeding may start at this time
Vital signs	Some change in BP from anesthesia (lower) or medications (higher), pulse may be slower, temperature may be slightly elevated for 24 hour

PHYSICAL ASSESSMENT

The physical assessment of the neonate is head-to-toe and involves the following components and anticipated findings:

COMPONENT	ANTICIPATED FINDINGS
Posture (at rest)	Flexed extremities, clenched fists
Body/Muscle tone	Resists extension of extremities (assessed throughout)
Moro Reflex	Response to loud sound, loss of support
Vital Signs	
Temperature	97-99° axillary
Heart rate	120-160 bpm (at rest) 160-180 bpm (crying) 80-120 bpm (deep rest)
Respiratory rate	30-60 rpm >60 rpm (crying)
Vital statistics	
Weight	2500-4000 grams (5 lb 8 oz - 8 lb 13 oz) <2748 grams (SGA or preterm) >4000 grams (LGA)
Length	18-22 inches (45-55 cm)
Head circumference	12.5-13.75 inches (32-35 cm)
Chest circumference	2 cm less than head circumference

COMPONENT	ANTICIPATED FINDINGS
Abdominal circumference	Approximately the same as chest
Skin	
Color	Pink or consistent with ethnicity
Lanugo	Amount (decreases with gestational age)
Turgor	Elastic
Head	
Molding	Overlapping suture lines present
Anterior fontanelle	Diamond shape (3-4 cm × 2-3 cm)
	Depressed in dehydration
	Bulging in intracranial pressure
Posterior fontanelle	Triangle shape (0.5-1.0) cm)
Hair	Fine, color
Face	Symmetry of features and movement
	Eyebrows and eyelashes present
Eyes	Blue, slate gray
	White sclera
	PERRLA, red reflex, blink reflex

COMPONENT	ANTICIPATED FINDINGS
Mouth	Epstein's pearls
	Intact hard and soft palate
	Uvula midline: Root, suck, swallow, gag, extrusion reflexes
Nose	Nares patent (obligatory nose breather)
Milia	Present on face (bridge of nose, chin)
Ears	Symmetric
	Top in line with eye canthi
	Hearing (responds to sounds)
Head lag	45° or less
Neck	
Mobility	Full range of motion
Thyroid gland	Nonpalpable
Lymph nodes	Nonpalpable
Clavicles	Intact
Control	Raises head when supine
	Brief control in erect position
Reflex	Tonic neck
Chest	
Shape	Cylindric, symmetric
Expansion	Symmetric, synchronous with abdomen

COMPONENT	**ANTICIPATED FINDINGS**
Auscultation	Lung sounds CTA (clear to auscultation)
	Heart sounds, rate, regular
PMI	Palpable & observable at 4th interspace
Breast	Palpable bud (5-10 mm)
Brachial pulses	Palpable, equal bilaterally
	Equal with PMI

Abdomen

Shape	Round, symmetric
Umbilicus	2 arteries, 1 vein
	No protrusion
Auscultation	Bowel sounds present @ 1-2 hours of life
Palpation	Slight diastasis recti
	Liver edge (@-1 cm below costal margin)
	Spleen (@-1 cm below left costal margin)
	Kidneys
Percussion	Liver, spleen size
Femoral pulse	Palpable equal bilaterally
	Equal with PMI

COMPONENT	ANTICIPATED FINDINGS
Genitalia	
Urination	First voiding within 24 hours of age
Labia	Majora > or cover minora
Vagina	Vaginal tag Mucous and or bloody discharge
Penis	Meatus at tip Foreskin adherent to glans
Scrotum	Rugae, testes descended
Back and Anus	
Buttocks	Symmetrical
Spine	Straight, flexible
Alignment	Shoulders, scapulae, & iliac crests
Sacrum	Intact
Reflexes	Trunk incurvation, crossed extension Landau
Anus	Patent Meconium, transitional stools Wink reflex
Extremities	
Arms	Symmetry of movement Flexed at rest Equal length Moro reflex response Palmar grasp

COMPONENT	ANTICIPATED FINDINGS
Hands	Fingers separate, 5 each hand
	Finger nails present
	Palmar crease normal
Legs	Symmetry of movement
	Flexed at rest
	Equal length, symmetric skin folds
	Ortolani maneuver (no dislocation or clicks)
	Stepping reflex
Feet	Plantar sole creases
	5 separate toes each foot
	Plantar grasp
	Babinski reflex

ASSESSMENT OF GESTATIONAL AGE

Assessment Component	Value	Criteria
Posture at rest	0	Extension of all extremities
	1	Extension of arms
		Beginning flexion of thighs
	2	Extension of arms
		Beginning flexion of legs
	3	Beginning flexion of arms, flexion of legs
	4	Complete flexion of arms and legs
Square Window	0	90° angle
		(Hypothenar eminence & forearm)
	1	60° angle
	2	45° angle
	3	30° angle
	4	0° angle

Assessment Component	Value	Criteria
Arm recoil	0	Arms remain extended
	1	Not applicable
	2	100-180° angle (at elbow)
	3	90-100
	4	<90° degree angle
Popliteal angle	0	180° angle (extension)
		(angle behind the knee)
	1	160° angle
	2	130° angle
	3	110° angle
	4	90° angle
	5	<90° angle
Scarf sign	0	Elbow at opposite arm
	1	Elbow at opposite shoulder
	2	Elbow at opposite nipple
	3	Elbow at midline

Assessment Component	Value	Criteria
Scarf sign	4	Elbow at same side nipple
Heel to ear	0	Toes touch ear, 180° angle (behind knee)
	1	Toes almost touch face
		130° angle
	2	110° angle
	3	90° angle
	4	90° angle
Physical maturity Skin	0	Edematous extremities,
		Color red
		Skin transparent
	1	Tibial edema
		Smooth pink color
		visible veins
	2	No edema
		Superficial peeling and/or rash
		Few veins

Assessment Component	Value	Criteria
Physical maturity **skin**	3	
		Cracking
		Pale areas
		Rare veins
	4	Deep cracking
		Parchment-like skin
		No veins
	5	Cracked, wrinkled leathery
Lanugo	0	None
	1	Abundant
	2	Thinning
	3	Bald areas
	4	Mostly bald
Plantar crease	0	None
	1	Faint red marks (upper ½ sole)
	2	Anterior transverse crease only
	3	Creases over anterior ⅔ of sole
	4	Creases cover entire sole

Assessment Component	Value	Criteria
Breast	0	Nipple barely perceptible
		No palpable breast bud
	1	Nipple present
		Flat areola
		No palpable breast bud
	2	Stippled areola with flat edge
		1-2 mm breast bud
	3	Stippled areola with raised edge
		3-4 mm breast bud
	4	Full areola & 5-10 mm breast bud
Ear	0	Pinna flat (no cartilage) soft remains folded
	1	Slightly curved pinna, soft slow recoil (unfolding)
	2	Well curved pinna, soft ready recoil

Assessment Component	Value	Criteria
Ear *(continued)*	3	Formed pinna, firm to edge
		Instant recoil
	4	Thick cartilage, ear stiff
Genitals: **Male**	0	No testes in scrotum, no rugae present
	1	Not applicable
	2	Testes descending, few rugae
	3	Testes within scrotum, good rugae
	4	Testes in pendulous scrotum, rugae cover scrotum
Female	0	Prominent clitoris and labia minora
	1	Not applicable
	2	Labia majora & minora equally prominent

Assessment Component	Value	Criteria
Female *(continued)*	3	Labia majora appear large, labia minora appear small
	4	Labia majora completely cover labia minora

TOTAL SCORE: _____

MATURITY RATING

Determined by comparing the total score with the corresponding weeks gestation according to the following values

TOTAL SCORE	WEEKS GESTATION
5	26
10	28
15	30
20	32
25	34
30	36
35	38
40	40
45	42
44	50

HIV PRETEST COUNSELING

PRE-TEST COUNSELING

1. Assist patient in evaluating risk.
    Since 1983 have you:

    Had sex without a condom?

    Used IV drugs? Shared needles?

    Had a blood transfusion of any kind?

    Had a job in which you were exposed to blood, such as with a needle stick?

    Been in any country where HIV is epidemic?

    Had or been exposed to a sexually-transmitted disease?

    Had sex with anyone who has been in jail or prison?

2. The pros and cons of testing:

    - If results negative, emotional relief from fear, can take steps to protect self in future
    - If results positive,
    - Able to take steps to decrease symptoms of AIDS
    - Prophylactic medications can "buy time" for curative medicines to be discovered
    - Can take steps to prevent infection of others
    - Can help with personal decision making in other ways. For example, the test results could help a person decide whether or not to have a baby.

Disadvantages of positive test

Emotional trauma of:

- Knowing AIDS is always fatal
- Living with uncertainty
- Being known as an infected person and/or person with AIDS with potential for social isolation, harassment
- Recognizing that the disease causes physical pain
- Knowing that personal relationships may be threatened
- Knowing that employment may be threatened
- Knowing potential for transmission to baby if pregnancy occurs
- Fear of infecting others if life-style changes not made
- May perpetuate risk behaviors

3. Acknowledge that decision to be tested is difficult, that recognition of risk for a life-threatening illness is involved.

4. Describe procedure:
   - Blood draw
   - Advise of time period required to obtain results.
   - Explain that positive results are confirmed with a second test, usually another kind of test.
   - Explain reasons for requiring test results to be given in person.

5. Discuss the reliability of the test. ELISA is 99% sensitive and specific.

6. Explain the meaning of a negative test.

- Not exposed to HIV
- Lag time for development of antibody (6 to 52 weeks)
- Possible need to be retested.

7. Explain the meaning of a positive test. The HIV positive person is infected and is infectious but does not have AIDS.

8. Explain the differences between anonymous and confidential testing. (Confidential testing restricts test results to the medical file.)

9. Ask patient if more information or time is needed to make a decision.

10. Review ways to avoid exposure.

11. Explain that help will be given to arrange counseling and medical evaluation if test results are positive.

12. Ask how she generally deals with stress/crisis and how she thinks she might deal with learning she is HIV positive.

13. Make an appointment for a follow-up meeting to discuss test results. Discuss the potential for stress/ anxiety during this period.

HIV POST - TEST COUNSELING: NEGATIVE RESULTS

Inform that result is negative. Show client lab result form:

1. Review what a negative test means:

- The body showed no signs of HIV.

- If exposure has been recent *(within the last 6 months)* the body may not yet show signs of infection. Therefore, repeat test in 6 months.

2. Explore client's response to negative test result:

   - Determine if there is ongoing risk of exposure
   - Review modes of transmission:
     - Sexual contact
     - Blood/blood product ingestion as with sharing needles
     - Perinatal transmission

3. Provide new information as appropriate about:

   - Safer sex
   - Safer use of drugs

4. Instruct on current selection and application of condoms:

   - Explore feeling about their use.
   - "Have you ever used a condom?"
   - "What was your experience with using them/How do you feel about them?"
   - "Have you ever talked about condoms with your partner?"
   - Demonstrate proper use using a model and encouraging client to touch the condom. Be playful; talk about new ways to make love.
   - Explore which condoms might be best for this client.
   - Discuss condom lubrication, price, and community resources for free condoms.

- Conduct strategy session that includes a discussion of ways to negotiate with partner for safer sex behaviors.

- Inquire about possible need for partner to come in for counseling/testing.

- Encourage commitment to staying negative.

- Emphasize the need for ongoing testing in association with at-risk behavior.

- Give HIV literature if acceptable to client and appropriate reading level literature is available (Remember that half of US adults read at or below the 9th grade level and most health education materials are written above the 9th grade level. This information is cited in a useful book titled, *Teaching Patients with Low Literacy Skill* by Cecilia Dosk and Leonard Dosk. It is published by Lippincott.)

HIV POST-TEST COUNSELING
POSITIVE RESULT

1. Make sure the room is private and quiet. Arrange for no interruptions; allow plenty of time. The client may remember little of what is said. Be patient. Be prepared for shock, denial, anger, confusion, anxiety. Consider the advantages of having two counselors present to provide support.

2. Inform that test is positive. Hand the client the lab report so that the results are seen.

3. Determine the client's understanding of what a positive test means.

4. Review the correct meaning of the antibody test as needed

   - Infection with HIV
   - Lifelong infection until treatment/cure discovered
   - At risk status for AIDS

5. Review the reliability of the test, if appropriate.

6. Acknowledge the reasonableness of fear of suffering or dying or repeated losses (physical strength, mental acuity, sexual freedom, self sufficiency and possibly family, lovers, friends, a job). Do not minimize the gravity of the client's situation. Do not attempt to assess time frame for development of AIDS.

7. Discuss client's support systems within own social network and/or support groups. Make a referral to a support group if appropriate.

8. Explain spectrum of disease if client seems able/ready to hear. Speak with realistic optimism. Avoid use of the word "victim."

9. Emphasize the importance of a medical evaluation as soon as possible so that a baseline evaluation can be made and prophylactic medication started. Emphasize the importance of a health care provider who has experience with PWAs. Make referral if possible.

10. Assess possibility of pregnancy.

11. If in the childbearing years and not using birth control and/or desirous of pregnancy, encourage to

postpone pregnancy until a knowledgeable decision can be made.

12. Begin process of assessing client's willingness to notify contacts. If the client is ready to do this, help her plan how it will be done. Key points include a private setting, anticipation of anger/blame, need for testing, and importance of safer sex/safer use.

13. Encourage the client to think a while before deciding whom else to tell. Rehearse ways to tell others if appropriate.

14. Discuss advisability of testing for potentially infected family members.

15. Emphasize the importance of attention to good health habits including avoiding alcohol, cigarettes, marijuana, and drugs as well as the positive benefits of sleep and good food.

16. Stress the importance of keeping insurance policies up to date.

17. Discuss the continuing importance of following safer sex and safer use guidelines to avoid infecting others, to minimize chances for repeated exposure to the virus, and to avoid exposure to other STDs with consequent strain on the immune system.

18. Remind not to donate blood, plasma or body organs. Do not breast feed. Do not share toothbrushes, safety razors or other items that could have blood on them.

19. If appropriate, discuss need for/possible consequences of sharing results with sexual partners, relatives, friends, school, health care providers.

20. Offer literature if deemed appropriate. Be sure that any material given is at an appropriate reading level. Explore with the client what might happen if the material were to found by others.

22. Evaluate the potential for suicide.

23. Give phone numbers or office callback and AIDS crisis or information hot lines.

24. Schedule a follow-up counseling appointment within a few days.

UNIVERSAL PRECAUTIONS AGAINST AIDS

- Practice careful handwashing, before and after wearing gloves.
- Wear gloves when coming into contact with body fluid, mucous membranes, or open wounds.
- Wear gloves when handling items soiled by blood and body fluids.
- Wear gloves when skin is broken or compromised.
- Wear gloves when starting IVs and drawing blood.
- Place needles, sharps, and scalpels in designated needle box.
- Needles are not cut and are not recapped.
- Empty needle box regularly to avoid overfilling
- Clean up blood or body fluids with 1:20 solution of Clorox and water. This solution should be prepared daily in order to hold its strength.
- Wear masks, gowns and goggles when involved in procedures that might produce splashes of blood or body fluids.

- Place all soiled linen in the appropriate isolation containers.
- Beware of the dangers of blood and body fluids, whether a patient has been diagnosed with AIDS or not.

ISOLATION PROCEDURES

Isolation, techniques prevent dissemination of harmful pathogens to susceptible patients and/or health care workers by establishing barriers to these pathogens. The Center for Disease Control issues recommendations for isolation procedures; however, hospitals will establish their own protocols for following these recommendations. Therefore, nurses may see wide variances in how the guidelines are implemented.

ASSESSMENT

- ❖ Physicians's orders and agency policy
- ❖ Medical diagnosis
- ❖ Isolation required

EQUIPMENT

- ❖ Private room with door closed at all times
- ❖ Door sign with isolation level
- ❖ Linen gown
- ❖ Disposable gowns, masks, gloves, caps, goggles, and shoe covers
- ❖ Separate laundry hamper
- ❖ Waste container with plastic lining
- ❖ Antimicrobial soap

- Disposable, sterile utensils, dishes, tray
- Sterile linen, diagnostic tools, or any articles that will contact patient
- Isolation labels
- Preparation
- Wash hands and examine for breaks in skin
- Identify patient
- Assemble equipment
- Explain precautions and procedures to patient, family, and visitors
- Place isolation sign and instructions on door.

PROCEDURES

- For infected patient: Gown gloves, and mask according to isolation level. Elevate bed to working level. Carry out intended procedure or care of patient.
- Provide appropriate containers for disposal of materials. Avoid vigorous movement of bed linen.
- Dispose of all waste items including gloves, mask and paper gowns before leaving room.

RATIONALE

- Protects nurse from contamination
- Receives isolation materials
- Prevents dissemination of pathogens by area movement
- Contaminated items may not leave room until properly disposed

PROCEDURES

With second nurse standing outside of room holding clean cuffed plastic bag, first nurse securely fastens plastic lined bag containing contaminated material. Red labels identify contents. Nurse outside room holds second bag open and first bag is drop inside second bag

- ❖ Remove gowns before leaving room.

- ❖ Wash hands before untying gown ties

- ❖ Remove gown inside out and roll up

- ❖ Before entering room, using strict medical asepsis, wash hands

RATIONALE

- ❖ "Double bagging" decreases possibility of contamination to environment outside of patient's room.

- ❖ Prevents transportation of pathogens.

- ❖ Prevents spread of microorganisms.

- ❖ Area of gown touching uniform is considered clean By rolling, harmful pathogens are trapped inside.

ISOLATION LEVELS

Strict

Private room, gown, masks, gloves when entering, all articles in room considered contaminated. Use disposable dishes. Prevents dissemination by contact and airborne sources. Recommended most commonly in childhood diseases. Rarely used except for varicella (chicken pox), Zoster (shingles), smallpox, and diphtheria.

Respiratory

Private room, mask when in close contact with patient. Double bag linens and trash. All articles in room considered contaminated. Prevents dissemination by contact and airborne sources. Infections requiring respiratory isolation include measles, epiglottitis, meningitis, pneumonia, mumps, whooping cough (pertussis).

Enteric

Private room, gown and gloves if handling articles with feces and vomitus. Infection may spread by direct or indirect contact. Prevents dissemination by contact with contaminated articles or feces. Common infections requiring enteric isolation are amebic dysentery, cholera, diarrhea of unknown cause, encephalitis, Hepatitis A, viral meningitis and gastroenteritis.

Blood/body Fluid

Private room, gown and gloves if handling articles contaminated with blood or body fluids. Prevents dissemination by direct or indirect contact with blood or body fluids. Double bag linens and trash. Common infections requiring this isolation are AIDS, Hepatitis B and C, malaria and syphilis.

Body Substance

Instituted in 1987, this procedure requires masks, gloves, gowns and goggles. It is a protection against any body substance, including sweat and tears. It has largely replaced respiratory isolation.

AFB (Acid Fast Bacilli)

This is a new, highly-specialized isolation that recommends special ventilation of rooms and protective clothing. It focuses on preventing the spread of tuberculosis.

Wear gown and masks if in direct contact: gloves are not necessary. Double bag linens and trash.

Drainage/Secretion

Gown, gloves when handling drainage or secretion from any source. Prevents dissemination by contaminated articles. This procedure is not widely used because it has been incorporated into the blood/body fluid guidelines. Infections include draining wound infections such as abscess, minor burns, decubitus ulcers and conjunctivas.

Contact

Private room, gown, mask, gloves for anyone in contact with patient. All articles in contact with patient are considered contaminated. Prevents dissemination by contact and airborne sources. This is the next most strict isolation. Rarely used except in methicillin resistant infections. Infections requiring this isolation are diphtheria, some cases of influenza, impetigo, pediculosis(lice),staph or strep pneumonia, rabies, rubella,and scabies

Note:Protective or reverse isolation is not an official CDC category. However, physicians may order it on an individualized basis, especially for oncology patients. All levels require labeling and bagging of contaminated materials.

TEACHING TOPICS

TEACHING TOPICS

PROBLEMS OF PREGNANCY AND INTERVENTIONS

First trimester

Problem: Nausea, vomiting ("morning sickness")

Interventions:

Dry crackers, toast in AM; frequent, small meals; avoid offensive odors; eliminate highly-seasoned fried food liquids with meals.

Problem: Malnutrition (obesity/underweight)

Interventions:

Provide dietary lists of food inclusions to ensure adequate nutrition in pregnancy and weight gain of 25-30 pounds, provide reduction calories in overweight while maintaining nutrients; monitor weight gain.

Problem: Breast changes (soreness/enlargement)

Interventions:

Wear supportive bra night and day; expose nipples to air qd for ½ hour; avoid trauma, strong soaps.

Problem: Leukorrhea, excessive perspiration

Interventions:

Daily shower with mild soap, use deodorant, wear cotton undergarments, apply light dusting of cornstarch to genitalia.

Problem: Urinary frequency
Interventions:
Maintain close proximity to bathroom, wear protective pad/undergarment.

Problem: Leg cramps, varicose veins
Interventions:
Reduce intake of calcium-rich foods; exercise by walking; elevate/extend legs when sitting; position foot in dorsiflexion; avoid standing in one place for long periods of time, crossing legs, wearing garters

Problem: Vertigo, headaches
Interventions:
Monitor BP for elevation, position on left side when lying down, change position slowly.

Problem: Fatigue
Interventions:
Rest periods during day, use of relaxation techniques.

Problem: Nasal stuffiness, epistaxis
Interventions:
Avoid blowing nose hard, provide humidification, avoid nasal/decongestion sprays, lower head, apply ice to back of neck or apply pressure to nose if bleeding occurs.

Problem: Dyspareunia

Interventions:

Teach that decreased interest in sexual activity and responsiveness are normal; suggest position changes that might decrease discomfort.

Problem: Use of drugs, alcohol, smoking

Interventions:

Teach hazards of these practices or conditions; risk of sexually transmitted diseases to the fetus; refer to counseling, treatment, rehabilitation.

Second trimester:

Problem: Chloasma ("mask of pregnancy"), striae gravidarum, body shape changes

Interventions:

Teach that these changes are normal, suggest clothing and makeup that will enhance appearance.

Problem: Backache

Interventions:

Teach pelvic lift exercises, suggest wearing low-heeled shoes, avoid belts/restrictive clothing.

Problem: Inadequate exercise

Interventions:

Teach body mechanics and correct posture, importance of walking; suggest sit-ups, squatting, stretch/press exercises, walking posture; Kegel's exercises.

Third trimester:

Problem: Edema (dependent/generalized)

Interventions:

Avoid constrictive clothing, sitting or standing for long periods of time, monitor I&O; elevate feet when sitting, assume side-lying position for sleep, avoid adding salt to foods; maintain comfortable room temperature.

Problem: Difficulty breathing

Interventions:

Use pillows to elevate head and chest for sleep, avoid eating large meals, teach good posture, breathing changes are normal.

Problem: Pyrosis, bloating, flatulence

Interventions:

Avoid gas-forming, greasy/fried foods, hot/cold foods; teach to eat small meals more frequently; maintain upright position during and after eating; chew gum; suck hard candy; suggest antacid if approved by physician.

Problem: Constipation, hemorrhoids

Interventions:

Dietary inclusion of fiber; fluid intake 8-10 glasses/day; walking/exercises within limits; stool softener as prescribed; avoid laxatives/ enemas; provide sitz baths; topical anesthesia ointment to anal area; using gloved finger, reinsert hemorrhoids as needed.

Problem: Sleep disturbance, insomnia

Interventions:

Suggest naps during the day, positions for sleep using pillows for support, warm shower, reading, relaxation exercises before H.S.

Problem: Urinary frequency

Interventions:

Reduce fluid intake before H.S., avoid prolonged upright/supine positions, maintain proximity to bathroom.

Problem: Anxiety about labor, welfare of infant

Interventions:

Teach stages of labor, contraction characteristics and timing, differences between Braxton-Hicks contractions and those indicating labor.

Postpartum

Problem: Involution

Interventions:

Teach that uterine fundus decreases in size qd after initial 48 hour until normal size occurs in 4-6 weeks; massage fundus to maintain tone, maintain urinary elimination to prevent bladder distention.

Problem: Pain ("after pains")
Interventions:

Mild analgesic as prescribed, teach that pain occurs in multigravida and increases in severity with increased number of births.

Problem: Lochia
Interventions:

Teach that rubra (bright red) is present for 2-4 days, serous (brownish) 4-6 days, then alba (yellowish-white); report excessive or foul-smelling lochia.

Problem: Urinary retention
Interventions:

Monitor I&O, suggest voiding q3h, allow water to run, pour warm water over genitalia, encourage to void during shower if urge present, fluid intake of 6-8 glasses/day, catheterize only if needed, perform Kegel's exercises.

Problem: Episiotomy, hemorrhoids
Interventions:

Apply ice pack, cleanse from front to back after elimination, change pad after each elimination; provide moist heat (sitz bath) after 24-48 hours, 2-4 times per day, provide dry heat (heat lamp) for 20 minutes, 2 times /day, local anesthesia ointment, spray, compresses to area, teach positions for sitting to avoid discomfort.

Problem: Breast engorgement

Interventions:

Apply ice pack, wear supportive bra, avoid actions that stimulate nipples, teach breast and nipple care if nursing (cleansing, air exposure, use of nursing pads, application of ointment, use of heat lamp, use of breast pump).

Problem: Postpartum depression

Interventions:

Allow expression of feelings, teach and support abilities to care for infant, teach that feeling depressed is normal after birth, provide privacy for nonverbal expression of feelings (crying, irritability, mood changes) involve in planning care for infant, monitor for signs of postpartum psychosis, refer to counseling if needed.

Problem: Weight loss

Interventions:

Inform of usual weight loss after birth (about 17 pounds); provide weight reduction diet if overweight, taking into consideration lactation.

EPISODIC HISTORY

Episodic history assessments are made at each prenatal visit. The episodic history includes a summary of physical and emotional problems and complaints since the previous prenatal visit. Specific questions can be asked based on expected needs of each trimester. The following is a sample list by trimester:

FIRST TRIMESTER

Discomforts

- Breast changes
- Fatigue
- Nausea and/or vomiting
- Nasal stuffiness and/or epistaxis
- Family dynamics
- Gingivitis
- Leukorrhea
- Psychosocial responses

Self-Care

- Exercise
- Rest and relaxation
- Nutrition

Warning or Danger Signs

- Bleeding
- Chills and fever
- Persistent, severe vomiting
- Burning on urination
- Cramping diarrhea

SECOND TRIMESTER

Discomforts

- Faintness
- Gastrointestinal distress
- Neuromuscular distress
- Psychosocial responses
- Skin changes
- Family dynamics
- Gingivitis
- Palpitations
- Skeletal distress
- Varicosities

Self-Care

- Exercise
- Rest and relaxation
- Nutrition
- Sexuality

Warning or Danger Signs

- Bleeding
- Chills and fever
- Decreased or absent fetal movements
- Ruptured membranes
- Burning on urination
- Diarrhea
- Persistent, severe vomiting

THIRD TRIMESTER

Discomforts
- Ankle edema
- False labor
- Fatigue
- Insomnia
- Perineal pressure
- Psychosocial responses
- Dizziness
- Family dynamics
- Gingivitis
- Leg cramps
- Shortness of breath
- Urinary frequency

Self-Care
- Baby preparation
- Labor preparation
- Rest and relaxation
- Exercise
- Nutrition
- Sexuality

Warning or Danger Signs
- Bleeding
- Chills and fever
- Epigastric pain
- Preterm labor
- Severe headache
- Burning on urination
- Diarrhea
- Generalized edema
- Rupture of membranes
- Visual disturbances

WELL-BEING ASSESSMENTS

Well-being assessments of the mother and fetus involve physical assessment, laboratory tests, and fetal growth data collection. The purpose is to document pregnancy growth and development and to identify potential problems early. The following assessments are made during each prenatal visit:

Physical Assessment:

- Maternal weight gain
- Maternal vital signs
- Fetoscope auscultation from 19 or 20 weeks to birth
- Fetal heart rate (120-160 bpm)
- CVA tenderness
- Edema
- Doppler auscultation from 10 or 12 weeks to 20 weeks
- Homan's sign

Laboratory Tests:

- Hemoglobin and hematocrit (at 28 weeks)
- Urinalysis (each visit)

Fetal Growth and Development:

- Maternal serum alpha-fetoprotein (at 15-18 weeks)
- Quickening (date of maternal perception of first movement)
- Fetal presentation (from 32 weeks to birth)
- Fundal height (at each visit)
- Fetal movement (maternal report and examiner palpation)

SIGNS OF LABOR

Premonitory signs of labor occur several hours to several days before the onset of labor and act as an advanced warning or "premonition" that labor is impending. They signs include:

Lightening: The beginning of descent of the fetus into the pelvis. It occurs in primigravid mothers 2-3 weeks before the onset of labor and may not occur in multiparous mothers until sometime in the labor process.

Braxton-Hicks contractions: The irregular, intermittent, mild uterine contractions that have been occurring throughout pregnancy but were undetected by the expectant mother until near term. They become increasingly stronger until they cause maternal discomfort. Although they are frequently confused as the beginning of labor, they do not produce progressive change in the cervix, and they are, therefore, termed "false labor contractions".

Cervical changes: The cervix becomes softer, initial effacement, and initial dilation begin to occur a few days before the onset of labor.

Bloody show: Bloody show, which is noticed with passage of the mucous plug, consists of a small amount of blood mixed with mucous, and is pinkish in color. This sign usually occurs a few hours before the onset of labor.

Burst of energy: A few hours or days before the onset of labor. The mother suddenly feels very energetic and may be motivated to complete house cleaning, baking, and other activities previously omitted because of feelings of fatigue. The energy should be saved for labor.

Spontaneous rupture of membranes: A sudden gush of fluid escaping from the vagina which cannot be controlled by the mother. It can occur 12-24 hours before the onset of labor, or it may not occur until labor is well established

False Labor Signs

False labor signs are characteristics of uterine contractions that the expectant mother notices. However, the false labor contractions do not cause a progressive change in the cervix. The characteristics include the following:

- Contractions are irregular
- Pain is focused in the abdomen
- No significant change in duration, frequency, or intensity
- No change in cervical dilatation or effacement
- No change in intensity with walking

True Labor Signs

The true labor signs are characteristics of uterine contractions noticed by the expectant mother and when assessed by a health care provider are determined to cause progressive change (effacement and dilatation) in the cervix. The characteristics include the following:

- Contractions occur at regular intervals
- Duration of contractions lengthens
- Pain begins in back and radiates to abdomen
- Intensity strengthens
- Time between contractions pregressively shortens
- Intensity of contractions increases with walking
- Dilatation and effacement steadily progress

PAIN MANAGEMENT DURING LABOR

- ❖ Encourage relaxation and breathing techniques throughout labor.

- ❖ Encourage walking, especially during early labor.

- ❖ Allow mother to assume the position in which she feels more comfortable.

- ❖ Do not mention the word "pain." Speak in terms of progress, dilatation, and contractions.

- ❖ Use pillows for support when mother is lying down. She should not lie supine during labor because of the pressure this position puts on the major blood vessels.

- ❖ Offer backrub and encourage significant other to massage (especially effleurage and touch.)

❖ Offer ice chips, cold washcloths.

❖ Help mother conserve energy; do not ask unnecessary questions and "make conversation."

❖ Encourage mother to urinate frequently (a full bladder may slow descent of the fetus.)

❖ Keep mother informed of fetal position, station, fetal heartbeat, dilatation, and effacement.

❖ Encourage rest between contractions, even a nap if possible.

❖ Do not perform procedures during contractions.

❖ Provide emotional support to mother and significant other.

❖ Assess need for pain medication, especially during the transitional period.

THE BASIC FOUR FOOD PYRAMID GUIDE

FOOD GROUP	SERVINGS REQUIRED PER DAY	NUTRIENTS SUPPLIED
Dairy products	Adults, 2 to 3 servings	Protein, calcium vitamins A and D
Fruits and vegetables	5-9 servings including at least 1 serving of green or yellow vegetables and 1 serving of citrus fruit	Vitamin A and C; fiber*
Meat, fish, eggs, legumes	2 to 3 servings	Protein, iron, niacin, thiamin
Bread, cereal, grains	6-11 servings	Thiamin, niacin, complex carbohydrates

*Fiber is not a nutrient, but is essential in dietary intake

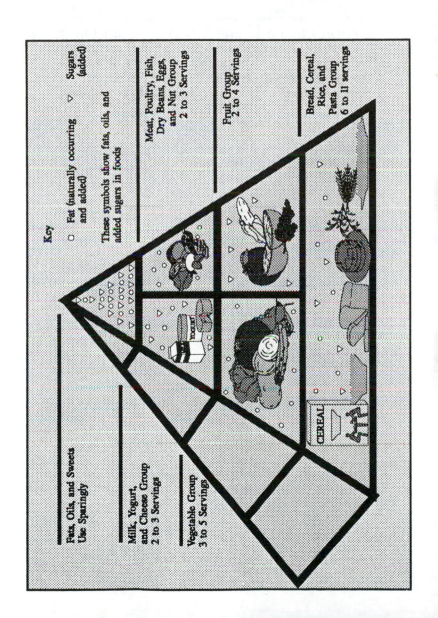

Key

○ Fat (naturally occurring ▽ Sugars
and added) (added)

These symbols show fats, oils, and
added sugars in foods

Fats, Oils, and Sweets
Use Sparingly

Milk, Yogurt,
and Cheese Group
2 to 3 Servings

Vegetable Group
3 to 5 Servings

Meat, Poultry, Fish,
Dry Beans, Eggs,
and Nut Group
2 to 3 Servings

Fruit Group
2 to 4 Servings

Bread, Cereal,
Rice, and
Pasta Group
6 to 11 servings

CEREAL

FOOD GROUP	SERVINGS DURING PREGNANCY	SERVINGS DURING LACTATION
Dairy Products	Four 8-oz cups	**Four 8-oz cups**
Milk Cheese Yogurt Cottage cheese Ice cream	1 cup milk = 1 ½ oz cheese 1 c. yogurt 1 ½ c.cottage cheese 1 ½ c. ice cream	
Meat Group	**Three servings**	Three servings
Beef Pork Poultry Fish Eggs Legumes Nuts Seeds Peanut butter	1 serving = 2 oz 1 serving = ½ c. legumes 1 T. peanut butter 1 egg	
Grain Products	Four servings	**Four servings**
Breads Cereal Pasta Rice	1 serving = 1 slice bread ¾ c. or 1 oz cereal ½ c. pasta ½ c. rice	

Fruits and Vegetables	Two to three servings	Two to three servings

Leafy green vegetables; deep yellow vegetables:
   Carrots
   Sweet potatoes
   Squash
   Tomatoes
Green vegetables
   Peas
   Green beans
   Broccoli
   Beets
   Cabbage
   Potatoes
   Corn
	(At least one serving of dark green or deep yellow vegetable for vitamin A)
	One serving = $\frac{1}{2}$ - 1 c. vegetable, 2 tomatoes, 1 medium potato	

Fats*	**One serving**	**One serving**
Butter Cream Nuts Cream cheese Avocadoes Oil	One serving = 1 tsp butter 2 T. cream 1 oz. cream cheese 1 med. avocado	

*Although fats are not officially a food group, they are essential because they supply Vitamins A and D and essential fatty acids, especially linoleic acid.

RECOMMENDED DAILY
ALLOWANCES FOR WOMEN

	15-18 Yr	19-24 Yr	25-50 Yr
Energy (kcal)	2,200	2,200	2,200
Protein (gm)	44	46	50
Vitamin A (μg RE)	800	800	800
Vitamin D (μg)	10	10	10
Vitamin E (mg α-TE)	8	8	8
Vitamin K (μg)	55	60	65
Vitamin C (mg)	60	60	60
Thiamin (mg)	1.1	1.1	1.1
Riboflavin (mg)	1.3	1.3	1.3
Niacin (mg NE)	15	15	15
Vitamin B_6 (mg)	1.5	1.6	1.6
Folate (μg)	180	180	180
Vitamin B_{12} (μg)	2	2	2
Calcium (mg)	1,200	1,200	800
Phosphorous (mg)	1,200	1,200	800
Magnesium (mg)	300	280	280
Iron (mg)	15	15	15
Zinc (mg)	12	12	12
Iodine (μg)	150	150	150
Selenium (μg)	50	50	50

RECOMMENDED DIETARY ALLOWANCES FOR PREGNANT AND LACTATING WOMEN

	Pregnant	LACTATING	
		1 st 6 mos.	2nd 6 mos.
Energy (kcal)	+ 0 1st tri +300 2nd tri +300 3rd tri	+500	+500
Protein (gm)	60	65	62
Vitamin A (µg RE)	800	1,300	1,200
Vitamin D (µg)	10	10	10
Vitamin E (mg α-TE)	10	12	11
Vitamin K (µg)	65	65	65
Vitamin C (mg)	70	95	90
Thiamin (mg)	1.5	1.6	1.6
Riboflavin (mg)	1.6	1.8	1.7
Niacin (mg NE)	17	20	20
Vitamin B_6 (mg)	2.2	2.1	2.1
Folate (µg)	400	280	260
Vitamin B_{12} (µg)	2.2	2.6	2.6
Calcium (mg)	1,200	1,200	1,200
Phosphorous (mg)	1,200	1,200	1,200
Magnesium (mg)	320	355	340
Iron (mg)	30	15	15
Zinc (mg)	15	19	16
Iodine (µg)	175	200	200
Selenium (µg)	65	75	75

Nutrient	Food Sources	Major Function
Protein	Complete protein from animal sources: Cheese Meat Milk Fish Poultry Eggs Incomplete protein (from plant sources): Peas Beans Rice Bread Cereal Nuts Complementary protein: Eggs and toast Cornbread and milk Beans and rice Spaghetti and meat sauce	Builds and maintains all body tissues; Builds blood; Aids in formation of antibodies; Provides energy after carbohydrates and fat supplies are exhausted

Nutrient	Food Sources	Major Function
Carbohydrates (Complex)	Breads Cereals Rice Pasta Potatoes Corn Fruits Vegetables	Body's major source of energy; Helps body utilize other nutrients
(Simple)	Sugar Honey, cookies Cake, pie Candy	
Iron	Red meats Cereal, especially Malt-o-Meal Oatmeal Apricots, Clams Prunes Liver Beans Baked potatoes Rice Spaghetti Almonds Wheat germ Spinach	Required for RBC reproduction; Heme in iron required for proper O_2-carrying RBCs; Required in pregnancy related to marked increase in blood volume; Prevents iron-deficiency anemia

Nutrient	Food Sources	Major Function
Vitamin A	Beef liver Sweet potatoes Carrots Spinach Cantaloupe Apricots Broccoli Asparagus Cheese	Maintains healthy skin, hair, mucous membranes; Repairs tissue, especially epithelial cells; Aids in bone growth and teeth development; Helps body resist infection; Essential for RNA reproduction and synthesis
Vitamin B$_1$ (Thiamin)	Poultry Pork Liver Milk Potatoes Breads Cereals Eggs	Essential for maintenance of circulation, digestion and nervous system; Maintains metabolic functions

Nutrient	Food Sources	Major Function
Vitamin B$_2$ (Riboflavin)	Beef liver Milk Steak Ricotta cheese Cottage cheese Spinach Brewer's yeast Broccoli Salmon Turkey	Essential for formation of RBC's and antibodies; Assists in metabolic function; Aids in building nerve structures; Helps cells to utilize oxygen
Vitamin B$_6$ (Pyridoxine)	Meat Liver Whole grains Beans Milk Bananas Prunes	Maintains antibody function; Essential for RNA and DNA synthesis; Critical for hemoglobin production; Helps maintain sodium and potassium balance; Balances nervous system function; Aids in tryptophan conversion

Nutrient	Food Sources	Major Function
Vitamin B$_{12}$ (Cobalamin)	Beef Eggs Milk Fish Pork	Essential for blood cell formation; Maintains healthy nervous system; Aids in iron absorption; Helps to maintain healthy appetite
Vitamin C	Orange juice Citrus fruits Broccoli Strawberries Green peppers	Essential for collagen production; Assists in bone and teeth formation; Essential for healing processes; Essential in RBC formation; Aids in resistance to infections

Nutrient	Food Sources	Major Function
Vitamin D	Egg yolk Liver Milk Salmon Tuna Sunlight	Necessary for absorption of calcium; Maintains healthy skin, hair, mucous membranes; Essential for formation of bones; Aids in maintaining balanced nervous system; Plays a role in blood clotting mechanisms
Vitamin E	Butter Eggs Fruit Nuts Oil Wheat germ Vegetables	Maintains integrity of muscles and nerves; Acts as an antioxidant in protecting other nutrients, especially Vitamins A and C; Specific role during pregnancy is not known
Vitamin K	Liver Oatmeal Green, leafy vegetables	Essential for coagulation of blood

Nutrient	Food Sources	Major Function
Folic acid	Eggs Milk Liver Seafood Green, leafy vegetables Whole grains Legumes Orange juice Wheat germ	Maintains cell growth and reproduction; Essential for RBC formation; Essential for DNA production; Aids in protein metabolism
Niacin	Eggs Lean meat Milk Poultry Seafood Whole grains	Aids in circulation; Aids in growth of body tissues; Maintains metabolism; Essential in sex hormone production
Phosphorus	Meat Fish Poultry Nuts Cheese Whole grains Phosphates in processed food	Maintains bones and teeth; Regulates heart beat; Assists in maintaining kidney function; Pairs with calcium

Nutrient	Food Sources	Major Function
Sodium	Table salt Soy sauce Seafood Cured meats Cheese Processed foods	Maintains fluid balance; Aids in functioning of nerves and muscles
Potassium	Meat Bran Potatoes Broccoli Bananas Peanut butter Green, leafy vegetables	Regulates heartbeat; Works with sodium to maintain fluid balance; Stimulates nerve impulses
Zinc	Shellfish Meat Liver Eggs	Maintains growth of sexual organs; Essential for production of enzymes; Aids in healing processes
Fats	Butter Yolks Fat in meat Bacon Milk Eggs Nuts	Supplies secondary source of energy; Supplies essential fatty acids, especially linoleic acid

Nutrient	Food Sources	Major Function
Calcium	Milk Cheese Salmon Sardines Nuts Beans	Essential for formation of bones and teeth; Maintains blood clotting mechanisms; Regulates heartbeat; Plays a role in growth of muscle tissue

RECOMMENDATIONS FOR NUTRIENT SUPPLEMENTATION DURING PREGNANCY

Supplement	Amount/Day	Indications
Iron*	30 mg	All pregnant women during 2nd and 3rd trimesters
Folate*	300 mcg	Pregnant women with inadequate intake of dietary folate
Multivitamin/mineral Preparation*		
Iron	30 mg	Pregnant women with inadequate diets or in high-risk categories such as multiple pregnancy, heavy cigarette smoking, or alcohol/ drug abuse
Zinc	15 mg	
Copper	2 mg	
Calcium	250 mg	
Vitamin B$_6$	2 mg	
Folate	300 mcg	
Vitamin C	50 mg	
Vitamin D	5 mcg	
Vitamin D	10 mcg (400 IU)	Complete vegetarians and women with low intake of Vitamin D-fortified milk

Supplement	Amount/Day	Indications
Calcium**	600 mg	Pregnant women under age 25 whose normal dietary intake is less than 600 mg/day
Vitamin B$_{12}$	2 mcg	Complete vegetarians
Zinc and Copper	15 mg 2 mg 30 mg/day	Women taking therapeutic iron supplementation

Taken between meals or at bedtime on empty stomach

**Taken at mealtime*

APPROXIMATE CAFFEINE CONTENT OF 1 CUP (8OZ) OF BEVERAGE

Beverage	Caffeine, mg
Coffee: Brewed	75-150
Coffee: Instant	30-80
Tea	40-60
Cola	30-60
Cocoa	2-40

FOOD SOURCES OF NUTRIENTS

Potassium-Rich Foods

- Avocados
- Broccoli
- Dried fruits
- Lima beans
- Navy beans
- Peaches
- Prunes
- Sunflower seeds
- Tomatoes
- Bananas
- Cantaloupe
- Grapefruit
- Nuts
- Oranges
- Potatoes
- Rhubarb
- Spinach

High-Sodium Foods

- Barbecue sauce
- Butter/margarine
- Canned seafood
- Cured meats
- Canned spaghetti sauce
- Buttermilk
- Canned chili
- Canned soups
- Dry onion soup mix
- Baking mixes (pancakes, muffins)

"Fast" Foods

- Macaroni and cheese
- Parmesan cheese
- Potato salad
- Sauerkraut
- TV dinners
- Microwave dinners
- Pickles
- Pretzels, potato chips
- Tomato ketchup

Calcium-Rich Foods

- Bok choy
- Cheese
- Cream soups
- Canned salmon/sardines
- Molasses (blackstrap)
- Broccoli
- Clams/Oysters
- Spinach
- Tofu
- Milk/ice cream

Vitamin K-Rich Foods

- Asparagus
- Broccoli
- Cabbage
- Cheeses
- Fish
- Mustard greens
- Rice
- Turnips
- Beans
- Brussel sprouts
- Cauliflower
- Collards
- Milk
- Pork
- Spinach
- Yogurt

Low-Sodium Foods

- Canned pumpkin
- Egg white and yolk
- Fruit
- Honey
- Lean meats
- Red kidney/lima beans
- Puffed wheat/rice
- Unsalted nuts
- Cooked turnips
- Fresh vegetables
- Grits (not instant)
- Jams and jellies
- Macaroons
- Baked/broiled poultry
- Sherbet
- Potatoes

Iron-Rich Foods

- Cereals
- Dried fruit
- Red meats
- Leafy green vegetables
- Dried beans
- Organ meats
- Peas

Foods that Acidify Urine

- Breads (whole grain)
- Cheeses
- Eggs
- Meats
- Poultry
- Cereals
- Cranberries
- Fish
- Plums
- Prunes

Foods that Alkalinize Urine

- All fruits except cranberries, prunes, plums
- All vegetables
- Milk

Foods Containing Tyramine

- Aged cheeses
- Bananas
- Bologna
- Chocolate
- Over-ripe fruit
- Yeasts
- Smoked or pickled fish
- Avocados
- Beer
- Caffeine
- Liver
- Red wine
- Yogurt

COMPLICATIONS OF PREGNANCY AND TREATMENTS

PROBLEMS WITH THE PLACENTA

Abruptio placentae (premature separation of a normally implanted placenta) or placenta previa (abnormal implantation of the placenta in the lower uterine segment near or over the cervical os) are most often the cause of latter pregnancy hemorrhage. The following chart lists the symptoms of these two complications of pregnancy:

Symptoms of Abruptio Placentae

- ❖ Absent to severe pain
- ❖ Concealed or obvious bleeding
- ❖ Dark red blood if obvious
- ❖ Bleeding continuous if obvious
- ❖ Uterine tone normal to boardlike
- ❖ Fetal position normal
- ❖ Fetal position abnormal
- ❖ Shock absent to severe
- ❖ PIH common
- ❖ Coagulopathy occasional to common
- ❖ History of trauma, hypertension or cocaine use and previous abruptio placentae

Nursing Interventions

- ❖ Infuse IV, prepare to administer blood
- ❖ Type and crossmatch
- ❖ Monitor FHR
- ❖ Insert Foley
- ❖ Measure degree of hemorrhage; count pads or weigh Chux (1g = 1 ml blood)
- ❖ Report signs/symptoms of DIC
- ❖ Monitor vital signs for shock
- ❖ Strict I&O
- ❖ Monitor CVP
- ❖ Provide supportive therapy in an emergency situation

Symptoms of Placenta Previa

- ❖ No pain
- ❖ Small to heavy bleeding
- ❖ Bright red blood
- ❖ Increase in fundal height due to bleeding
- ❖ No increase in fundal due to bleeding
- ❖ Normal uterine tone
- ❖ Bleeding intermittent
- ❖ Shock (occasional)
- ❖ PIH not usual
- ❖ Coagulopathy rare

Nursing Interventions

❖ Bedrest

❖ Prepare to induce labor if cervix is ripe

❖ Prepare for Cesarean birth

❖ Vital signs every four hours

❖ Type and crossmatch in case blood is required

❖ Administer IV

HYPEREMESIS GRAVIDARUM

Hyperemesis gravidarum is excessive nausea and vomiting of pregnancy resulting in electrolyte, nutritional, and metabolic imbalances. Possibly caused by elevated estrogen levels and the higher HCG levels of the first trimester, especially increased with multiple gestation and hydatidiform mole, the disorder is often corrected with restoration of the imbalances and completion of the first trimester. With proper intervention, the outcome is essentially the same as for pregnancies without hyperemesis gravidarum. If the imbalances are not corrected, however intrauterine growth retardation, CNS malformations, and embryonic/fetal death may be the outcome for the neonate.

Symptoms of Hyperemesis Gravidarum

❖ Vomiting of all intake

❖ Retching between oral intake

❖ Dehydration

❖ Fluid and electrolyte imbalances

❖ Hypotension

❖ Tachycardia

- Increased hematocrit and BUN
- Oliguria
- Metabolic acidosis
- Weight loss
- Jaundice
- Starvation

Nursing Interventions

- Administer fluids, at least 3000 ml/day
- Monitor strict I&O
- When oral intake is allowed, provide 6 small meals with plenty of liquids
- Administer Phenergan IM for nausea and vomiting
- NPO for first 48 hours

PREGNANCY-INDUCED HYPERTENSION

PIH (Pregnancy-Induced Hypertension), is a disorder characterized by hypertension, proteinuria, and edema. PIH is classified as mild or severe preeclampsia based on severity of symptoms, as eclampsia when convulsions occur, and as HELLP (Hemolysis, Elevated Liver enzymes, and Low Platelet count) Syndrome when preeclampsia and eclampsia have increased in severity.

Symptoms of PIH

Mild preeclampsia:

- Hypertension (increase of 30/15 mm Hg or more)
- Proteinuria ("trace" to 1+ by dipstick)
- Edema (dependent plus puffiness of fingers and face)

❖ Reflexes (3+ but no clonus)

❖ Weight gain (1 lb/week)

Severe Preeclampsia:

❖ Hypertension (160/110 mm Hg or more)

❖ Proteinuria (2+ or greater by dip stick)

❖ Edema (generalized, pulmonary edema)

❖ Reflexes (3+ or greater with ankle clonus)

❖ Weight gain (1 lb/week; may be sudden increase)

❖ Oliguria

❖ Severe headache

❖ Visual disturbances (blurred, photophobia, spots)

❖ Severe irritability

❖ Epigastric pain

❖ Elevated serum creatinine

❖ Thrombocytopenia

❖ AST markedly elevated

❖ Increased hematocrit (hemoconcentration)

Eclampsia:

❖ Symptoms of severe preeclampsia

❖ Convulsions

HELLP syndrome:

❖ Symptoms of PIH

❖ AST and ALT elevated

❖ Platelet count (low)

❖ BUN elevated

❖ Creatinine elevated

Nursing Interventions

Preeclampsia:

❖ Diet high in protein (80g/day)(to replace protein in urine)

❖ Bedrest

❖ Administer magnesium sulfate for convulsions

❖ Be prepared to administer calcium gluconate as an antidote, if required.

❖ Moderate sodium intake

❖ Monitor FHR

❖ Daily weight

❖ Monitor deep tendon reflexes

❖ Monitor LOC to note impending convulsion

❖ Left lateral position (to decrease pressure on vena cava and increase general circulation)

❖ Monitor fetal movement

❖ Be prepared to administer diazepam (Valium) as a sedative

❖ Administer hydralazine (Apresoline) to lower blood pressure (has no adverse effect on fetus)

❖ Monitor breath sounds

❖ Observe q hr for vaginal bleeding

❖ Provide psychological support

Commonly-Administered Medications
- ❖ Magnesium Sulfate (antidote is Calcium Gluconate)
- ❖ Fluid and electrolyte replacement
- ❖ Valium or phenobarbital as sedatives
- ❖ Apresoline (antihypertensive).

Medications Administered as Tocolytics
- ❖ Magnesium Sulfate
- ❖ Terbutaline
- ❖ Yutopar

EDEMA
- ❖ Edema is evaluated to differentiate between the expected dependent edema of pregnancy and generalized edema which would indicate the potential for development of PIH during labor.

- ❖ If generalized edema is present, deep tendon reflexes would also be assessed for further signs of PIH.

ECTOPIC PREGNANCY

Ectopic pregnancy occurs when gestation takes place outside the uterus—often in the ampullar or isthmus section of the fallopian tube. Ectopic pregnancy is the second leading cause of death of pregnant women in the United States.

Symptoms of Ectopic Pregnancy

Unruptured:

- ❖ Missed period
- ❖ Early symptoms of pregnancy
- ❖ Abdominal pain within 3-5 weeks of missed period (may be generalized or one-sided)
- ❖ Vague discomfort
- ❖ Scant, dark brown vaginal bleeding
- ❖ Positive serum pregnancy test

Tubal rupture:

- ❖ Syncope
- ❖ Use of IUD
- ❖ Abdominal cramping
- ❖ Shoulder pain (indicative of intraperitoneal bleeding that extends to diaphragm and phrenic nerve)
- ❖ Sudden, sharp, severe pain
- ❖ Use of oral contraceptives
- ❖ Signs of hypovolemic shock:
- ❖ Hypotension
- ❖ Tachycardia

❖ Tachypnea

❖ Cullen's sign (blue tinge around umbilicus)

Nursing Interventions

❖ Vital signs

❖ Administer IV fluids (especially for shock)

❖ Monitor for vaginal bleeding (Strict I&O)

❖ Monitor signs/symptoms of hypovolemic shock

The Puerperium

Developmental Changes of the Puerperium

The developmental changes of the puerperim involve the taking-in phase, the taking-hold phase and the letting-go phase. The characteristics of each of summarized below:

Characteristics of the taking-in-phase:

❖ Passivity

❖ Dependence on others

❖ Low energy level

❖ Difficulty in making decisions

❖ Reliving labor and birth experience

❖ Focus more on self than on infant

❖ Phase lasts one to three days in primigravida, perhaps only a few hours in multigravida

Characteristics of the taking-hold phase:

- ❖ Independent
- ❖ Increased energy level
- ❖ Initiates self-care activities
- ❖ Assumes increasing responsibility for neonate's care
- ❖ Receptive to education for self-care and infant-care
- ❖ Eager to provide "right" infant care
- ❖ Easily loses confidence in ability to care for infant
- ❖ Increased focus on infant
- ❖ Emotional support required to set realistic goals

Characteristics of letting-go phase:

- ❖ Interdependence between mother and other family members
- ❖ Acceptance of real child; gives up fantasy child
- ❖ Retains, roles, characteristics and relationships compatible with new role as mother
- ❖ Lasts throughout growing years

Maternal Comfort Measures:

Perineal comfort measures

Nonpharmacologic therapy

- ❖ Use of ice during first 24 horus
- ❖ Heat (whirlpool, sitz bath), 12-24 hours postpartum

❖ Kegel exercises

Pharmacologic therapy

❖ Administration of analgesic medication (usually oral)

❖ Application of anesthetic sprays PRN

Hemorrhoid comfort measures

❖ Use of ice

❖ Heat (whirlpool, sitz bath)

❖ Use of sidelying position

❖ Inflatable ring

❖ Tucks

Pharmacologic therapy

❖ Anesthetic ointment or suppository

❖ Stool softeners

❖ Avoiding prolonged sitting

Abdominal comfort measures

❖ Lying in prone position

❖ Ambulation

❖ Warm bath

❖ Use of analgesic medication (one hour before breastfeeding for lactating mother to promote comfort)

Breast engorgement comfort measures

Lactating mother

- ❖ Early initiation of breastfeeding
- ❖ Supportive bra
- ❖ Warm shower
- ❖ Warm packs/ice packs

Nonlactating mother

- ❖ Breast binder/supportive bra
- ❖ Ice packs
- ❖ Mild analgesic

Muscular comfort measures

- ❖ Backrubs
- ❖ Comfortable positioning
- ❖ Warm bath
- ❖ Mild analgesia

Rest measures

- ❖ Providing periods of uninterrupted rest
- ❖ Transferring telephone calls to nurses station while mother rests

Sleep measures

- ❖ Scheduling maternal assessments during infant feeding times to avoid frequent sleep interruption

❖ Assisting mother in assuming position of comfort

❖ Providing backrub

❖ Relieving sources of discomfort (perineal, abdominal, breast)

Physiologic Well-being Measures

❖ Uterine involution

❖ Prevention of uterine atony due to distended bladder

❖ Remind mother to empty bladder often

❖ Use fundal massage to stimulate uterine contraction

❖ Administer oxytocin for persistently atonic uterus (to halt excessive blood loss)

Perineal hygiene

❖ Changing perineal pad with each voiding

❖ Use of surgigator with each voiding and bowel movement

❖ Wiping from front to back after voiding or a bowel movement

Breast care

Nonlactating mother

❖ Support bra for first week (bottle-feeding mother)

Lactating mother

❖ Support bra

❖ Avoiding stimulation of the breast

❖ Avoiding warm shower water falling directly on breasts

❖ Use of ice packs to prevent engorgement

❖ Use of mild analgesia for engorgement discomfort

Elimination measures

❖ Reminding mother to empty bladder often

❖ Administration of stool softener once or twice daily to promote bowel elimination

❖ Catheterization if mother is unable to void

Nutrition measures

❖ Adequate fluid intake to support lactation

❖ Diet which promotes tissue healing

❖ Bowel elimination

❖ Sufficient calories

Maternal Self Care Measures

Perineal Self-care

❖ Change perineal pad after each voiding or bowel movement

❖ Wipe from front to back after elimination

❖ Apply perineal pad to the front first

❖ Avoid tampons until placental site is healed

Breast self-care
❖ *Lactating mother*
  - Avoid soap on nipples (causes dyring/cracking)
  - Use nonplastic backed breast pads (plastic holds in moisture/causes growth of bacteria)
  - Wear supportive bra
  - Keep nipples dry

❖ *Nonlactating mother*
  - Supportive bra for one week
  - Avoid breast stimulation
  - Complete lactation suppression medication as prescribed

Afterpain self-care
  - ❖ Lying in prone position
  - ❖ Ambulation
  - ❖ Warm bath
  - ❖ Use of analgesic medication (one hour before breastfeeding for lactating mother to promote comfort)

Elimination self-care
  - ❖ Fluid intake (8-10 glasses of water per day)
  - ❖ Roughage in diet

❖ Perineal self-care information

Nutrition self-care

❖ Balanced meals high in protein and Vitamin C to promote tissue healing

❖ Roughage from fresh fruits and vegetables to prevent constipation

Rest self-care

❖ Information about resting or napping in morning and afternoon

Exercise self-care

❖ Gradually resuming daily activities

❖ Performing postpartum exercises as instructed by health care provider

Sexual activity self-care

❖ Use of nonsexual intercourse intimacy until episiotomy site and placental site have healed

❖ Placental site is considered healed when lochia discharge has ceased (about 3 weeks)

❖ Vagina will be dry because of decreased level of estrogen

❖ Use of water-soluble lubricant will make intercourse more comfortable

❖ Breastfeeding before sexual intercourse will reduce leaking due to sexual stimulation in lactating mother

Immunizations self-care

❖ Avoid pregnancy for three months following rubella vaccine

❖ Need to administer RhoGAM following each birth or abortion for Rh negative mother

INFANT CARE MEASURES

Educating the parent for infant care involves providing information on and demonstration of daily care activities based on individual parental education needs. Education for the new parents should include the following points:

❖ Handling (cradle, upright, football hold)

❖ Positioning (side-lying after feeding)

❖ Feeding

❖ Burping

❖ Nasal and oral suctioning

❖ Bathing (sponge bath until cord falls off)

❖ Tub bathing (baby is slippery)

❖ Umbilical cord care (keep it dry)

❖ Signs of umbilical cord infection

❖ Nail care

- Swaddling/wrapping
- Dressing (1 light layer of clothing more than the parent has)
- Taking temperature (axillary preferred)
- Voiding
- Stools (consistency, color, number for breastfed infants)
- Diapering
- Sleep
- Activity
- Crying
- Circumcision care
- Safety (car seat)
- Screening tests
- Immunizations

Guidelines For Calling Health-care Provider for Infant

- Temperature (100.4 degrees F. axillary; 97.8 degrees F. axillary or less)
- Frequent vomiting over a period of time (6 hours)
- Loss of appetite (refused 2 successive feedings)
- Blue skin color (especially lips)
- Difficult to awaken (lethargy)

❖ Apnea (15 seconds)

❖ Bleeding or discharge from any opening

❖ Diarrhea (2 or more green, watery stools)

❖ Dehydration (<6 wet diapers in 24 hours, sunken anterior fontanelle)

❖ Continuous high-pitched cry

Information for Developmental Adjustment to Parenting Role

❖ Set priorities for tasks that need to be performed and identify priorities that can wait or can be done by others

❖ Avoid moving to a new location during the puerperium

❖ Avoid the temptation to perform exceptional housecleaning (identify housecleaning, cooking, laundry tasks that friends or family can perform)

❖ Schedule naps (morning and afternoon the first 1-2 weeks; unplug the phone, do not answer the door)

❖ Go to bed early

❖ Avoid accepting other responsibilities (care of extended family members, community projects, church activities)

❖ Schedule quiet time away from the baby and out of the house

❖ Schedule "couple time" between mother and father

- ❖ Select contraceptive method before first sexual activity
- ❖ Communicate openly with partner and others
- ❖ Include father in infant care activities
- ❖ Plan for infant day care and return to work
- ❖ Discuss with partner who will do what activities during puerperium and after mother returns to work

SUMMARY OF METHODS OF CONTRACEPTION

Contraceptives are used to prevent, plan or space pregnancies, of select the number of children desired and to controlthe timing of the birth of each child. Listed below is a summary methods available, advantages, disadvantages, side effects and contraindications for each method. Contraceptives are classified as oral contraceptives, spermicides, barrier methods, long-acting methods, voluntary sterilization and fertility awareness methods.

ORAL CONTRACEPTIVES AVAILABLE
IN THE UNITED STATES
Estimated Estrogen/Progestin Potency

Progestin: Intermediate
Estrogen: *Low*

- Demulen 1/35
- Lo/Ovral

- Levlen
- Nordette

Progestin: *Low*
Estrogen: *Low*

Monophasic:

- Bravicon
- Genora 1/35
- Loestrin 1/20
- Loestrin 1.5/30
- N.E.E. 1/35 E
- Nelova 1/35 E
- Norcept-E 1/35
- Norethin 1/50 M
- Norinyl 1 + 50
- Ortho-Novum 1/50

- Genora 0.5/35
- Genora 1/50
- Loestrin Fe 1/20
- Modicon
- Nelova 0.5/35 E
- Nelova 1/50 M
- Norethin 1/35 E
- Norinyl 1 + 35
- Ortho-Novum 1/35
- Ovcon-35

Biphasic

- Nelova 10/11

- Ortho-Novum 10/11

Triphasic

- Ortho-Novum
- Tri-Levlen
- Triphasil

- 7/7/7
- Tri-Norinyl

Progestin: High
Estrogen: Intermediate
- Ovral

Progestin: Intermediate
Estrogen: Intermediate
- Demulin 1/50
- Norlestrin Fe 2.5/50
- Norlestrin 2.5/50

Progestins: Low
Estrogens: Intermediate

Monophasic
- Norlestrin 1/50
- Ovcon 50
- Norlestrin 1/50

Achieving Hormonal Balances with Oral Contraceptives

Side Effects: Estrogen

Excess:
- Nausea
- Melasma
- Migraine headache
- Breast fullness/tenderness
- Bloating
- Hypertension
- Edema

Deficiency
- Early or midcycle breakthrough bleeding

- Increased spotting
- Hypomenorrhea

Side Effects: Progestin
Excess

- Increased appetite
- Fatigue, feeling tired
- Acne, oily scalp
- Depression
- Breast regression

- Weight gain
- Hypomenorrhea
- Hair loss, hirsutism
- Monilial vaginitis

Deficiency

- Late breakthrough bleeding
- Hypermenorrhea

- Amenorrhea

ESTROGEN-PROGESTIN CONTRACEPTIVES

Mode of Action: **Inhibits ovulation**

Effectiveness: **0.1%**

Advantages:

- Prevention of benign breast cysts and fibroadenomas
- Relief of problems associated with menstrual cycle (cramps, pain)
- Easily reversible
- Prevention of ectopic pregnancy

- Timing of next menses known
- Protection against ovarian and endometrial cancer
- Improvement of acne
- Suppression of functional ovarian cysts

- Method not associated with intercourse (spontaneity)
- Safety
- Protection against acute pelvic inflammatory disease

Disadvantages:

- Pill must be taken at same time daily
- Side effects
- Decreased effectiveness with other medications (*antibiotics, anticonvulsants*)
- Does not protect against STDs
- Expense
- Does not protect against HIV

Side Effects:

- Mood changes (in some women)
- Chloasma (in some women)
- Circulatory complications (rare)
- Nausea (with first packet or first few pills of each pack)
- Missed menses
- Breast fullness/tenderness (in some women)
- Headaches (in some women)
- Increased risk of liver tumors (rare)
- Spotting or breakthrough bleeding

Indications:

- Heavy or painful menses
- Recurrent ovarian cysts
- Family history of ovarian cancer
- Patient who desires spacing of pregnancies
- Acne
- Nulliparous women
- Sexually active young women/adolescents
- Nonlactating postpartal women

Contraindications:

- Breast cancer
- Diabetes
- Coronary artery disease
- Impaired liver function
- Current or past liver adenoma
- Cholestatic jaundice during pregnancy
- Surgery planned within 4 weeks
- Surgery/immobilization involving lower extremity

- Hypertension
- Current or past stroke
- Gallbladder disease
- Heavy smoker
- Past or current thromboembolism
- Sickle cell hemoglobinopathy
- Patient over 40 years age

PROGESTIN-ONLY CONTRACEPTIVE METHODS
Implants (norplant); injections

Mode of Action: **Inhibits ovulation**

Advantages:

- Highly effective
- Method not associated with intercourse (*spontaneity*)
- No estrogen-related side effects
- Decreased menses cramping and pain (in some women)

- Easily reversible
- Long-acting (*5 years for implant, 3 months for injection*)
- Scanty or no menses (*in some women*)
- Does not suppress lactation

Disadvantages:

- Injections required
- Implant may be slightly visible
- Amenorrhea (irregular menstrual cycle)

- Delayed reversal
- High initial expense for implant
- Minor surgery required to insert and remove implant

Side Effects:

- Menstrual irregularities

Indications:

- Continuous contraception
- Long-term spacing of births desired
- Patient does not want sterilization

- Lactation
- Patient does not desire more children
- Side effects have been experienced with other contraception methods

Contraindications:

- Acute liver disease
- Unexplained, undiagnosed vaginal bleeding
- Cardiac disease or cerebrovascular disease

- Jaundice
- Thrombophlebitis or pulmonary embolism

OTHER CONTRACEPTIVE METHODS

Spermicides: Chemical which kills sperm

Advantages:

- Over-the-counter availability
- Provide lubrication
- Can be used to backup other contraceptive methods
- Protection against some STDs
- Temporary method

Disadvantages:

- Method associated with intercourse
- Messy
- Typical failure rate of 21%

Side Effects:

- Skin irritation in some users

Indications:

- Need for backup method
- Need for method without prescription
- Temporary need

Contraindications:

- Vaginal abnormality which prevents correct placement and retention of spermicide in vagina to cover the cervix
- Allergy to ingredients
- Inability to use spermicide correctly

Barrier Methods: Condoms, diaphragm, sponge, cervical cap

Action: Mechanical barrier preventing transportation of the sperm to the ovum

Advantages:

- Inexpensive
- Accessible (over-the-counter availability)
- Health provider intervention not required (except for diaphragm and cap)
- Safe
- Protection against STDs
- Prevents messiness of seminal discharge in the vagina

Disadvantages:

- Method associated with intercourse
- Defective device

Side Effects:

- Skin irritation (in some users with some methods)
- Increased risk of urinary tract infections (diaphragm)
- Possibility of increased yeast infections (sponge)
- Difficulty removing sponge
- Pap smear abnormalities with cap
- Vaginal dryness (sponge)

Contraindications:

- Allergy to rubber, latex, polyurethane or chemicals
- Inability to learn correct insertion/application technique
- History of toxic shock syndrome
- Repeated urinary tract infections

Intrauterine devices (IUD)

Action: Not fully understood; may be due to effect on sperm, ova, fertilization, implantation, endometrium and/or fallopian tube

Advantages:
- Method not associated with intercourse
- Long-acting contraception

Disadvantages:
- Must be inserted and removed by health provider
- Increased menstrual bleeding (*in some women*)
- Dysmenorrhea (*in some women*)

Side Effects:
- Uterine/cervical perforation or embedding (*rare*)
- Expulsion (*during first year in some women*)
- Increased risk for pelvic inflammatory disease (*during first few weeks in some women*)

Indications:
- Monogamous relationships
- Multiparous women

Contraindications
- Pregnancy
- PID
- Absolute (*method not prescribed*)

Relative (*not prescribed unless other methods even less desirable*):
- Purulent cervicitis
- Recurrent gonorrhea
- Ectopic pregnancy history
- Impaired coagulation

- Undiagnosed irregular bleeding
- At risk for STD (*multiple partners/partner with multiple partners*)
- Postpartumor postabortion infection

Other relative (*prescribed with careful monitoring*):

- Valvular heart disease
- Menstrual disorder
- Uterine anomalies
- Anemia

Sterilization: Vasectomy (*men*) tubal ligation/blockage (*women*)

Action: Prevents ova transport through fallopian tube (*tubal ligation*) and prevents sperm transport through vas deferens (*vasectomy*)

Advantages:

- Permanent
- Safe
- Highly effective
- Economical

Disadvantages:

- Minor surgical procedure
- Irreversible

Indications:

- Personal preference
- Medical disorders
- Multiparity
- Hereditary disease

Contraindications:

- Youth (*under 21 years of age if federal funds involved*)
- Mental incompetence

Fertility Awareness Methods

Action: Abstinence from sexual intercourse during fertile period of menstrual cycle

Advantages:

- Safety
- Promote learning about body functions
- No religious objections
- No cost
- Useful to plan pregnancy

Disadvantages:

- Extensive abstinence for irregular menstrual cycles
- Extensive counseling to learn correct use of methods

Side Effects:

- Frustration during periods of abstinence

Indications:

- Personal or religious desire to use "natural" method; willingness to accept unplanned pregnancy

Contraindications:

- Irregular temperature chart results
- Unwillingness to use abstinence during fertile period
- Irregular menstrual cycles
- Anovulatory menstrual cycles
- Inability to keep accurate charts

CLINICAL VALUES
AND STANDARDS

CLINICAL VALUES AND STANDARDS

STANDARD LABORATORY VALUES: PREGNANT AND NONPREGNANT WOMEN		
	PREGNANT	**NONPREGNANT**
HEMATOLOGIC VALUES		
Complete Blood Count (CBC)		
Hemoglobin, g/dl	12-16*	10-14*
Hematocrit, PCV, %	37-47	32-42
Red cell volume, ml	1600	1900
Plasma volume,ml	2400	3700
Red blood cell count, million/mm^3	4-5.5	4-5.5
White blood cells, total per mm^3	4500-10,000	5000-15,000
Polymorphonuclear cells, %	54-62	60-85
Lymphocytes, %	38-46	15-40
Erythrocyte sedimentation rate, mm/h	$\leq$	30-90

* At sea level. Permanent residents of higher levels (e.g. Denver) require higher levels of hemoglobin.

STANDARD LABORATORY VALUES: PREGNANT AND NONPREGNANT WOMEN		
	PREGNANT	**NONPREGNANT**
MCHC, g/dl packed RBCs (mean corpuscular-hemoglobin concentration)	No change	30-36
MCH/(mean corpuscular hemoglobin per picogram [less than a nanogram])	No change	29-32
MCV/μm^3 (mean corpuscular volume per cubic micrometer)	No change	82-96
Blood coagulation and fibrinolytic activity†		
Factors VII, VIII, IX, X	Increase in pregnancy, return to normal in early puerperium: Factor VIII increases during and immediately after delivery	50% - 150% of normal
†Pregnancy represemts a hypercoagulable state		

STANDARD LABORATORY VALUES: PREGNANT AND NONPREGNANT WOMEN		
	PREGNANT	**NONPREGNANT**
Factors XI, XIII	Decrease in pregnancy	
Prothrombin time (protime)	Slight decrease in pregnancy	10-15 sec.
Partial thromboplastin time (PTT)	Slight decrease in pregnancy and again decrease during second and third stage of labor (indicates clotting at placental site)	60-70 sec.
Bleeding time	No change	1-5min (Duke) 1-9 min (Ivy)
Coagulation time	No change	6-10 min (Lee/White)

STANDARD LABORATORY VALUES: PREGNANT AND NONPREGNANT WOMEN		
	PREGNANT	**NONPREGNANT**
Platelets	No significant change until 3-5 days after delivery, then marked increase (may predispose woman to thrombosis) and gradual return to normal	150,000 to 350,000/mm^3
Fibrinolytic activity	Decreases in pregnancy, then abrupt return to normal (protection against thromboembolism)	
Fibrinogen	150-400mg/dl	450 mg/dl
MINERAL/VITAMIN CONCENTRATIONS		
Vitamin B$_{12}$, folic acid, absorbic acid	Moderate decrease	Normal

STANDARD LABORATORY VALUES: PREGNANT AND NONPREGNANT WOMEN		
	PREGNANT	**NONPREGNANT**
SERUM PROTEINS		
Total, g/dl	5.5-7.5	6.7-8.3
Albumin, g/dl	3.0-5.0	3.5-5.5
Globulin, total, g/dl	3.0-4.0	2.3-3.5
BLOOD SUGAR / GLUCOSE (Whole Blood)		
Fasting, mg/dl	≤ 90	70-105
2-hour postprandial, mg/dl	Under 140 after a 100 g carbohydrate meal is normal	70-120
CARDIOVASCULAR DETERMINATIONS		
Blood pressure, mm Hg	120/80*	114/65
Pulse, rate/min	70	80
Stroke volume, ml	65	75
*Value at 20 years of age ***For 30 years of age: 123/82** ***For 40 years of age: 126/84**		

STANDARD LABORATORY VALUES: PREGNANT AND NONPREGNANT WOMEN		
	PREGNANT	**NONPREGNANT**
CARDIOVASCULAR DETERMINATIONS (continued)	+	
Cardiac output, L/min		
Circulation time (arm-tongue), sec		
Blood Volume, ml		
Whole blood	5600	4000
Plasma	3700	2400
Red blood cells	1900	1600
CHEST X-RAY STUDIES		
Transverse diameter of heart	1-2 cm increase	—
Left border of heart	Straightened	—
Cardiac volume	70 ml increase	—
HEPATIC VALUES		
Bilirubin total	Unchanged	Not more than 1 mg/dl

STANDARD LABORATORY VALUES: PREGNANT AND NONPREGNANT WOMEN		
	PREGNANT	**NONPREGNANT**
Serum cholesterol	↑ 60% from 16-32 weeks of pregnancy; remains at this level until after delivery	110-200 mg/dl
Serum alkaline phosphate	↑ from week 12 of pregnancy to 6 weeks after delivery	2-4.5 units (Bodansky)
Serum globulin albumin	↑ slight ↓ 3.0 g by late pregnancy	1.5-3.0 g/dl 4.5-5.3 g/dl
	PREGNANT	NONPREGNANT
RENAL VALUES		
Bladder capacity	1500 ml	1300 ml
Renal plasma flow (RPF), ml/min	Increase by 25%, to 612-875	490-700
Glomerular filtration rate (GFR), ml/min	Increase by 50%, to 160-198	105-132

STANDARD LABORATORY VALUES: PREGNANT AND NONPREGNANT WOMEN		
	PREGNANT	**NONPREGNANT**
Nonprotein nitrogen (NPN), mg/dl	Decreases	25-40
Blood urea nitrogen (BUN), mg/dl	Decreases	5-20
Serum creatinine, mg/dl/24 hr	Decreases	0.5-1.1
Serum uric acid, mg/dl/24 hr	Decreases	2-6
Urine glucose	Present in 20% of gravidas	Negative
Intravenous pyelogram (IVP)	Slight to moderate hydroureter and hydronephrosis; right kidney larger than left kidney	Normal

Initial Prenatal Screening
CBC:

- Hemoglobin, g/dl
- Hematocrit, PCV,%
- Red cell volume, ml
- Plasma Volume, ml
- Red blood cell
  count, million/mm^3
- White blood cells,
  total per mm^3
- Polymorphonuclear
  cells, %
- Lymphocytes,%
- Erythrocyte
  sedimentationrate, mm/h
- MCHC, g/dl
  packed RBCs
  (mean corpuscular
  hemoglobin concentration)
- MCV/ μm^3
  (mean corpuscular volume
  per cubic micrometer)

Hepatic Tests

- Bilrubin total
- Serum cholesterol
- Serumalkaline phosphatase
- Blood type and RH Factor Rubella Titer antibody screen
- Seralogy urine culture and sensitivity
- Pap smear
- Gonorrhea and chlamydia screen
- Coombs for RH negative Molher
- Sickle cell screen for Black Mother

Successive Prenatal Laboratory Screening

- Urinalysis at each prenatal visit
- HCT and HGB at 24-28 weeks
- Glucose Screen at 24-28 weeks

High-Risk Population Prenatal Laboratory Screening

- HIV
- Hepatitis B
- HPV smear
- Hepatitis A
- Group B Streptococci
- Blood Smear
- Renal Function Tests: (BUN, creatinine, creatinine clearance, electrolytes, total protein excretion)
- Amniocentesis
- Amniotic fluid tests (alpha-fetoprotein L/S ratio, phosphatidylglycerol, creatinine)

Fetal Well-Being Screening in High-Risk Pregnancy:

- Amniocentesis
- Ultrasound
- Creatinine Level
- Chorionic Villus Sampling
- Percutaneous Umbilical Blood Sampling
- Lecithin/Sphingomyelin Ratio
- Alpha-fetoprotein
- Phosphatidylglycerol
- Biophysical Profile
- Nonstress Test
- Contraction Stress Test

Neonatal Well-Being Screening in High-Risk Pregnancy

- Cord Blood pH
- HCT
- Type and Rh
- Glucose
- HGB
- RBC
- Bilirubin

Screening for Complications of Childbearing

- RBC
- HCT
- Platelets
- Fibrinogen
- Prothrombin
- PTT
- Factors VII, VIII, IX, X
- HGB
- Blood Smear
- Blood Chemistry
- Fibrin Split Products
- PT
- Bleeding Time
- Factors XI, XIII

Renal Creatinine

- BUN
- Creatinine Clearance
- Uric Acid

Hepatic AST (SGOT)

- ALT (SGPT)
- Alkaline Phosphatase
- Bilirubin
- LDH
- Albumin

Thyroid Function Tests

LABORATORY VALUES IN THE NEONATAL PERIOD			
BLOOD VALUES	**TERM**	**NEONATAL**	**PRETERM**
Clotting factors:			
Activated clotting time (ACT)		2 min	
Bleeding time (Ivy)		1-8 min	
Fibrinogen		150-300 mg/dl	
Hemoglobin	17-19(g/dl)		15-17(g/dl)
Hematocrit	42-65(%)		45-55
Reticulocytes	3-7(%)		Up to 10
Fetal hemoglobin (% of total)	40-70		80-90
Clotting factor: Nucleated RBC/mm^3 (per 100 RBC)	200 (0.05)		(0.2)
Platelet count/mm^3	100,000-300,000		120,000-180,000
WBC/mm^3	15,000		10,000-20,000
Neutrophils (%)	45		47

LABORATORY VALUES IN THE NEONATAL PERIOD			
	TERM	**NEONATAL**	**PRETERM**
Eosinophils and basophils(%)	3		
Lymphocytes (%)	30		33
Monocytes (%)	5		4
Immature WBC (%)	10		16
OTHER CHEMISTRY			
Bilirubin, direct		0-1 mg/dl	
Bilirubin, total		Cord:< 2 mg/dl	
Peripheral: Total Bilirubin		1st Day: -6 mg/dl 2nd Day: -8 mg/dl 3rd-5thDay:-12 mg/dl	
Blood gases			
Arterial:		pH 7.31-7.45	
		Pco_2 50-80 mm Hg	

	TERM	NEONATAL	PRETERM
		Po$_2$ 50-70 mm Hg	
Venous:		pH 7.28-7.42	
		Pco$_2$ 38-52 mm Hg	
		Po$_2$ 20-49 mm Hg	
a1-fetoprotein		0	
Fibrinogen		150-300 mg/dl	

LABORATORY VALUES IN THE NEONATAL PERIOD

Urinalysis
Volume: 1-7 days, 20-40 ml daily
After the 1st week: 200 ml / 24 hours

Protein::present for2-4 days

Casts and WBCs: may be present in first 2-4 days

Osmolarity (mOsm/L): 100-600

pH: 5-7

Specific gravity: 1.001-1.020

LABORATORY VALUES IN THE NEONATAL PERIOD

CARDIOPULMONARY AND RESPIRATORY READINGS

Blood pressure:

Term: Systolic, 78 mm Hg; diastolic, 42 mm Hg

Preterm: Systolic, 50-60 mm Hg; diastolic, 30 mm Hg

Respiratory rate: 30-60 min

Fetal heart rate

Baseline: 120-160/min

Tachycardia: > 160 bpm (acceleratin may occur during uterine contractions)

Bradycardia: < 120 bpm

Early deceleration: Bradycardia with onset of contraction benign
Variable deceleration: Bradycardia due to cord compression; usually benign
Late deceleration: Bradycardia after lag period due to fetal hypoxia—ominous sign
Heart rate, term infant: 120-160 bpm

LABORATORY FINDINGS IN PREGNANCY			
RENAL VALUE:	**NONPREGANT**	**PREGNANT**	**PIH**
Renal Plasma flow Glomerular Filtration Rate BUN Serum Creatinie Serum Uric Acid	490-700 me/min 105-132 ml/ min 20-25 mg/dl 20-25 mg/dl 257-750 mg/kg 24 hr.	Increased U 612-875 25 R160-198 (50%) decreased decreased decreased	
Hematologic Values	Nonpregnant	Pregnant	PIH
Thrombocytopenia Hematocrit Platelets	Absent 37-47 % 150,000- 350,000/mm^3	Absent 32-42 % normal	PresentIncreased< 100,000/mm^3
Liver enzymes	Nonpregnant	Preganant	PIh
AST (SGOT) ALT (SGPT)	7-27 U/L 1-21 U/L	Normal Normal	Elevated Elevated

LABORATORY FINDINGS IN PREGNANCY

	Pre-Eclampsia:
BUN	< 80
Uric acid	< 5.0
Creatinine	< 0.8
Creatinine clearance	< 160
SGOT (IU/Liter)	< 11-32
Platelets	< 150,000
Fibrinogen	< 300-600
Hematocrit	< 40 *
Anemia	
Indices	
MCHC	32-37%
MCV	80-96/υ m^3
MCH	28-33/ picogram

LABORATORY FINDINGS IN PREGNANCY	
Reticular Count	0.5-1.5 %
Coagulation profile Pro time (sec) PTT (sec) IVY Bleeding Time (min) D Dimer Kleihauer-Betke (KB)	 10-11 < 40 2.5-9.5 < 0.5 < 0.1
Glucose (OHSU norms)	

1 Hr Screen (50 gram)
3 Hr GTT (100 Grams)
    Fasting
    1 Hr
    2 Hr
    3 Hr
* Depending on Baseline
	< 140 mg/dL
	
	105 mg/dL
	190 mg/dL
	165mg/dL
	145 mg/dL

WBC $\times 10^3$:	6.0 - 15.0
PMN (Neutrophils,"Segs," "Polys") Bands Lymphs Monos Eos Basophils	 60 - 85% 0 - 5% 21-45% 4 10% 1 - 5% 0 - 2%

LABORATORY FINDINGS IN PREGNANCY

Shift to left (elevated PMN and bands) = bacterial infection *if* WBC elevated

If WBC elevated, PMNs and bands are normal, and lymphs are elevated = viral infection

WBC up to 20,000 are normal in labor (stress response)

Chemistry	
NA+	136-145 mEq/L
K+	3.5-5.0 mEq/L
Cl	98-106 mEq/L
HCO$_3$	21-30 mEq/L

Iron Indices	
Serum Iron (micro gm/dl)	105± 35
TIBC	*360± 20
Percent Saturation	20-45%
Ferritin ng/ml	15-200
	*Higher due to estrogen

Folate Indices	
Serum Folate (ng/ml cells)	150-450
Vitamin B (pg/mλ)	200-600

LABORATORY FINDINGS IN PREGNANCY	
Liver Function Tests	
AST	7-27 U/L
SGOT (units/L)	11-32
LDH (units/L)	25-100
Bilirubin (mg/L)	0.3-1.0
Total	0.1-0.3
Direct	
Thyroid Function Tests	
Free T. (ng/100m)	1.1-2.1
TSH (micro units/m)	0.4-5.4
Thyroxine binding	10
Capcity(%)	

Previous use of oral thyroid medicine: order free T4

Enlarged thyroid and/or tachycardia and/or wide diastolic/systolic split: order free T4

Note: 99% of thyroxine is bound to protein; 1% is free and has end-organ effect, tachycardia and/or a wide split diastolic/systolic is found.

Common Abbreviations In Maternal-Newborn and Women's Health Nursing

ABC	*Alternative birthing center or airway, breathing circulation*
AC	*Abdominal circumference*
ACTH	*Adrenocorticotrophic hormone*
AFAFP	*Amnioticfluid alphafetoprotein*
AFP	*α–fetoprotein*
AFV	*Amniotic fluid volume*
AGA	*Appropriate for gestational age*
AID or AIH	*Artificial insemination donor (H designates mate is donor)*
AIDS	*Acquired Immune Deficiency Syndrome*
ARBOW	*Artificial rupture of bag of waters*
AROM	*Artificial rupture of membranes*
BAT	*Brown adipose tissue (brown fat)*
BBT	*Basal body temperature*
BL	*Baseline (fetal heart rate baseline)*
BMR	*Basal metabolic rate*
BOW	*Bag of waters*
BP	*Blood pressure*
BPD	*Biparietal diameter or Bronchopulmonary dysplasia*
BPM	*Beats per minute*
BSE	*Breast self-examination*
BSST	*Breast self-stimulation test*
CC	*Chest circumference or Cord compression*
cc	*cubic centimeter*
CDC	*Centers for Disease Control*

C-H	*Crown-to-Heel length*
CHF	*Congestive Heart Failure*
CID	*Cytomegalic inclusion disease*
CMV	*Cytomegalovirus*
cm	*centimeter*
CNM	*Certified nurse-midwife*
CNS	*Central nervous system*
CPAP	*Continuous positive airway pressure*
CPD	*Cephalopelvic disproportion or Citrate-phosphate-dextrose*
CPR	*Cardiopulmonary resuscitation*
CRL	*Crown-rump length of fetus*
C/S	*Cesarean section or C-section*
CST	*Contraction stress test*
CT	*Computerized tomography*
CVA	*Costovertebral angle*
CVP	*Central venous pressure*
CVS	*Chorionic villus sampling*
D&C	*Dilation and curettage*
decel	*deceleration of fetal heart rate*
DFMR	*Daily fetal movement response*
DIC	*Dissemination intravascular coagulation*
dil	*dilation*
DM	*Diabetes mellitus*
DRG	*Diagnostic related groups*
DTR	*Deep tendon reflexes*
ECHMO	*Extracorporal membrane oxygenator*
EDC	*Estimated date of confinement*
EDD	*Estimated date of delivery*
EFM	*Electronic fetal monitoring*

EFW	*Estimated fetal weight*
ELF	*Elective low forceps*
Epis	*Episiotomy*
FAD	*Fetal activity diary*
FAS	*Fetal alcohol syndrome*
FBD	*Fibrocystic breast disease*
FBM	*Fetal breathing movements*
FBS	*Fetal blood sample or fasting blood sugar test*
FECG	*Fetal electrocardiogram*
FFA	*Free fatty acids*
FHR	*Fetal heart rate*
FHT	*Fetal heart tones*
FL	*Femur length*
FM	*Fetal movement*
FMAC	*Fetal movement acceleration test*
FMD	*Fetal movement diary*
FPG	*Fasting plasma glucose test*
FRC	*Female reproductive cycle*
FSH	*Follicle-stimulating hormone*
FSHRH	*Follicle-stimulating hormone releasing hormone*
FSI	*Foam stability index*
G or grav	*Gravida*
GDM	*Gestational diabetes mellitus*
GI	*Gastrointestinal*
GnRH	*Gonadotrophin-releasing factor*
GnRH	*Gonadotrophin releasing hormone*
GTPAL	*Gravida, term, preterm, abortion, living children; a system of recording maternity history*

GYN	*Gynecology*
HA	*Head-abdominal rates*
HAI	*Hemagglutination-inhibition test*
HC	*Head compression*
hCG	*Human chorionic gonadotrophin*
hCS	*Human chorionic somatomammotropin (same as hPL)*
HMD	*Hyaline membrane disease*
hMG	*Human menopausal gonadotrophin*
hPL	*Human placental lactogen*
HVH	*Herpes virus hominis*
ICS	*Intercostal space*
IDDM	*Insulin-dependent diabetes mellitus (Type 1)*
IDM	*Infant of a diabetic mother*
IGT	*Impaired glucose tolerance*
IGTT	*Intravenous glucose tolerance test*
IPG	*Impedance phlebography*
IUD	*Intrauterine device*
IUFD	*Intrauterine fetal death*
IUGR	*Intrauterine growth retardation*
CCAH	*Joint Commission on the Accreditation of Hospitals*
LADA	*Left-acromion-dorsal-anterior*
LADP	*Left-acromion-dorsal-posterior*
LBW	*Low birth weight*
LDR	*Labor, delivery and recovery room*
LGA	*Large for gestational age*
LH	*Luteinizing hormone*
LHRH	*Luteinizing hormone-releasing hormone*

LMA	*Left-mentum-anterior*
LML	*Left mediolateral episiotomy*
LMP	*Last menstrual period or Left-mentum-posterior*
LMT	*Left-mentum-transverse*
LOA	*Left-occiput-anterior*
OF	*Low outlet forceps*
LOT	*Left occiput transverse*
L/S	*Lecithin/sphingomyelin ration*
LSA	*Left-sacrum-transverse*
MAS	*Meconium aspiration syndrome or Movement alarm signal*
MCT	*Medium chain triglycerides*
mec	*Meconium*
mec st	*Meconium stain*
M & I	*Maternity and Infant Care Projects*
ML	*Midline (episiotomy)*
MLE	*Midline echo*
MRI	*Magnetic resonance imaging*
MSAFP	*Maternal serum alpha fetoprotein*
MUGB	*4-methylumbelliferyl quanidnobenzoate*
multip	*Multipara*
NANDA	*North American Nursing Diagnosis Association*
NEC	*Necrotizing enterocolitis*
NGU	*Nongonococcal urethritis*
NP	*Nurse practitioner*
NPO	*Nothing by mouth*
NSCST	*Nipple stimulation contraction stress test*
NST	*Nonstress test or nonshivering thermogenesis*

NTD	*Neural tube defects*
NSVD	*Normal sterile vaginal delivery*
OA	*Occiput anterior*
OB	*Obstetrics*
OCT	*Oxytocin challenge test*
OF	*Occipitofrontal circumference*
OGTT	*Oral glucose tolerance test*
OM	*Occipitomental (diameter)*
OP	*Occiput posterior*
p	*para*
Pap smear	*Papanicolaou smear*
PBI	*Protein-bound iodine*
PDA	*Patent ductus arteriosus*
PEEP	*Positive end-expiratory pressure*
PG	*Phosphatidylglycerol or Prostaglandin*
PI	*Phosphatidylinositol*
PID	*Pelvic inflammatory disease*
PIH	*Pregnancy-induced hypertension*
Pit	*Pitocin*
PKU	*Phenylketonuria*
PMI	*Point of maximal impulse*
PPHN	*Persistent pulmonary hypertension*
Preemie	*Premature infant*
Primip	*Primapara*
PROM	*Premature rupture of membranes*
PTT	*Partial thromboplastin test*
PUBS	*Percutaneous umbilical blood sampling*
RADA	*Right-acromion-dorsal-anterior*
RADP	*Right-acromion-dorsal posterior*

REEDA	*Redness, edema, ecchymosis, discharge (or drainage) approximation (a system for recording wound healing)*
RDA	*Recommended dietary allowance*
RDS	*Respiratory distress syndrome*
REM	*Rapid eye movements*
RIA	*Radioimmunoassay*
RLF	*Retrolental fibroplasia*
ROA	*Right-occiput-anterior*
ROP	*Right-occiput-posterior*
ROP	*Retinopathy of prematurity*
ROM	*Rupture of membranes*
ROT	*Right-occiput-transverse*
RMA	*Right-mentum-posterior*
RMP	*Right-mentum-transverse*
RRA	*Radioreceptor assay*
RSA	*Right-sacrum-anterior*
RSP	*Right-sacrum-posterior*
RST	*Right-sacrum-transverse*
SET	*Surrogate embryo transfer*
SFD	*Small for dates*
SGA	*Small for gestational age*
SIDS	*Sudden infant death syndrome*
SOAP	*Subjective data,objective data, analysis, plan*
SOB	*Suboccipitobregmatic diameter*
SMB	*Submentobregmatic diameter*
SRBOW	*Spontaneous rupture of the membranes*
SROM	*Spontaneous rupture of the membranes*

STD	*Sexually transmitted disease*
STH	*Somatotrophic hormone*
STS	*Serologic test for syphilis*
SVE	*Sterile vaginal exam*
TC	*Thoracic circumference*
TCM	*Transcutaneous monitoring*
TNZ	*Thermal neutral zone*
TSS	*Toxic shock syndrome*
U	*Umbilicus*
u/a	*Urinalysis*
UA	*Uterine activity*
UAC	*Umbilical artery catheter*
UAU	*Uterine activity units*
UC	*Uterine contraction*
UPI	*Uteroplacental insufficiency*
U/S	*Ultrasound*
WBC	*White blood cell*

MEASUREMENT EQUIVALENTS

Metric System

1 Liter (L) = 1,000 milliliters (ml)

1 L. = 1,000 cubic centimeters (cc)

1 grain (gr) = 60 milligrams (mg)

1 mg = 1,000 micrograms (mcg)

1 gram (G) = 1,000 mg

1 cc = 1 ml

1 ounce (oz) = 30 G

1 ml = 16 minims (m)

2.5 centimeters (cm) = 1 inch (in)

1 kilogram (kg) = 1,000 G

1 kg = 2.2 pounds (lbs)

1 G = 1,000 kg

15 gr = 1 G

1 mcg = 0.001 mg

Apothecary

60 grains (gr) = 1 dram

8 drams = 1 ounce

16 ounces = 1 pint (pt)

60 minims = 1 dram

480 minims = 1 ounce

1 dram = 1 teaspoon (tsp)

4 drams = 1 tablespoon (tbls)

30 ml = 1 oz

Household

8 oz = 1 cup

1 teaspoon = 5 ml

1 glass = 240 ml

2 tablespoons = 1 oz

1 quart (qt) = 1,000 ml

1 pint = 500 ml

1 minim = 1 drop (gtt)

1 oz = 30 ml

1 pound = 16 oz

1 gallon = 4 quarts

1 quart = 2 pints

24 HOUR CLOCK

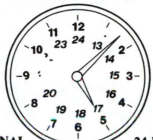

CONVENTIONAL 12 HOUR TIME	24 HOUR CLOCK TIME
12:01AM	0001
1:00 AM	0100
1:30 AM	0130
2:00 AM	0200
3:00 AM	0300
4:00 AM	0400
5:00 AM	0500
6:00 AM	0600
7:00 AM	0700
8:00 AM	0800
9:00 AM	0900
10:00 AM	1000
11:00 AM	1100
12 noon	1200
1:00 PM	1300
2:00 PM	1400
3:00 PM	1500
4:00 PM	1600
5:00 PM	1700
6:00 PM	1800
7:00 PM	1900
8:00 PM	2000
9:00 PM	2100
10:00 PM	2200
11:00 PM	2300
12 midnight	2400

DRUG ADMINISTRATION

DRUG ADMINISTRATION

DRUGS CONTRAINDICATED DURING BREAST FEEDING

- Meprobamate
  (Equanil)
- Diazepam *(Valium)*
- Ergot
- Heroin
- Chloramphenicol
- Reserpine

- Cyclophosphamide
  (Cytoxan)
- Diethylstilbestrol
- Gold
- Lithium
- Methotrexate

MEDICATIONS TO USE WITH CAUTION DURING BREASTFEEDING

- Aloe
- Barbiturates
- Depo-Provera
- Dihydrotachysterol
- Flagyl
- Isoniazid
- Norethindrone
- Phenylbutazone
- Senna
- Thiazides

- Atropine
- Chloral hydrate
- Dicumarol
- Ethinyl estradiol
- Indomethacin
- Methadone
- Phenothiazines
- Quinine
- Sulfonamides

COMMONLY USED MEDICATIONS
CONTAINING ASPIRIN

- Alka Seltzer

- Alka Seltzer Plus Cold Medicine

- Anacin

- Anacin Maximum Strength

- Arthritis Pain Formula

- Maximum Strength Midol for cramps

- Axotal

- BAC # 3

- BC Powder

- BC Tablets

- Buff-A-Comp

- Rid-A-Pain with Codeine

- Bufferin

- Cama Arthritis Strength

- Ascriptin

- Fiorinal #1, #2, #3

- Gemnisyn

- Lortab ASA

- Midol

- Excedrin

- Mepro-Analgesic

- Mepro Compound

- Norgesic

- Orphengesic

- P-A-C Tablets

- Buff-A-Comp # 3

- Robaxisal

- Soma Compound

- Cope

- Damason-P

- Duradyne

- Empirin # 2, #3, #4

- Equagesic

- Equazine-M

- Synalgos DC

- Talwin Compound

- Tecnal

- Trilisate

- Trigesic

- Vanquish

FDA Pregnancy Categories

A No risk demonstrated to the fetus in any trimester

B No adverse effects in animals, no human studies available

C Only given after risks to fetus are considered: animal studies have shown adverse reactions, no human studies available

D Definite fetal risks, may be given in spite of risks if needed in life-threatening conditions

X Absolute fetal abnormalities; not to be used anytime in pregnancy

DRUG ADMINISTRATION
COMMONLY USED MEDICATIONS

Generic	Trade	
Acetaminophen	Acephen	Neopan
	Anacin-3	Panadol
Classification:	Anuphen	Panex
Nonnarcotic analgesic	APAP	Paracetamol
Miscellaneous, antipyretic	(Atasol)	Pedric
	Banesin	
	(Campain)	(Robigesic)
	Datril	(Rounax)
Pregnancy Category B	Dolanex	St. Joseph's
	Genapap	Aspirin-Free
	Halenol	Suppap
	Liquiprin	Tempra
	Myapap	Tenol
	Nacetyl-P-	Tylenol
	aminophenol	Typap
		Ty-tabs

Comments

Available as: PO, Rectal

Used to treat: Mild to moderate pain, fever.

Implications: Assess pain or fever and response to medication. Give with 8 oz. of water. May be given with food or on an empty stomach. Do not give in malnutrition. Tylenol can cause severe liver damage when taken in large amounts over a prolonged period. Use cautiously in pregnancy and lactation. Warn patient against self medication for more than 10 days (adults) and 5 days (children)

Common side effects:

None significant. For overdose, acetylcysteine (mucomyst) is the antidote.

Generic
Bromocriptine

Trade
Parlodel

Classification
Ovulation stimulant

Pregnancy Category B

Comments
Available as: PO
Used to treat: Female infertility
Implications: Not to be used during pregnancy; may enhance
fertility in nonpregnant women. Monitor blood pressure (be sure
to get a baseline before administration). Administer with food or
milk to decrease GI distress.
Common side effects:
Dizziness, drowsiness, headache, insomnia, hypotension, nausea,
vomiting, anorexia.

Generic	**Trade**
Butorphanol	Stadol

Classification:
Narcotic Analgesic
Agonist / Antagonist

Pregnancy Category B

Comments
Available: IM, IV
Used to treat: Moderate to severe pain. Used during labor. Also used as a supplement to anesthesia.
Implication: Monitor pain relief. Closely monitor vital signs. When used during labor may cause respiratory depression in newborn. Do not use in undiagnosed abdominal pain. Chronic use can cause physical and psychological dependency.
Common side effects:
Sedation, headache, feeling of dysphoria, hypotension, nausea, diaphoresis.

Generic
Clindamycin hydrochloride

Trade
Cleocin

Classification:
Anti-infective

Pregnancy Category B

Comments
Available: PO, IM, IV, Topical
Used to treat: Respiratory tract infections, serious skin infections, gynecological infections.
Implications: Monitor CBC for decrease in WBC, platelets. Monitor for superinfection. Give PO with full glass of water. Give with meals. Do not refrigerate.
IV: Do not bolus undiluted. 1200-mg maximum in single IV infusion. Do not administer if crystals are present.
Common side effects:
Diarrhea, hypotension, phlebitis at IV site.

Generic	**Trade**
Clotrimazole	Gyne-Lotrimin
	Lotrimin
Classification:	Mycelex
Antifungal	

Pregnancy Category B

Comments

Available: PO, Topical, vaginal tablets, lozenges

Used to treat: Fungal infections, oropharyngeal and vaginal suppositories or cream are used in pregnancy candidiasis

Implications: Vaginal tablets for nonpregnant women only. Tell patient to allow lozenge to dissolve in mouth, do not swallow lozenge whole or chew.

Common side effects:

Nausea, vomiting, vaginal irritation (with tablets or cream).

Generic	**Trade**
Erythromycin	E-mycin, Erythromid RobimycinInclude s Erythromycin opthalmic ointment

Classification:
Antiinfective

Pregnancy Category B

Comments

Available: PO, IV, Topical Ophthalmic

Used to treat: Respiratory infections, streptococcal infections, chlamydia, syphilis, gonorrhea.

Implications: Monitor signs of infection, especially temperature. Crosses placenta and is found in breast milk. Erythromycin Estolate (estolate salt) is contraindicated in pregnancy. In the neonate, Ilotycin is used prophylactically for ophthalmic neonatorum, caused by *Neisseria gonorrhoeae* to prevent blindness. It is also used if the mother has been diagnosed with chlamydia.

Common side effects:

Nausea, vomiting, diarrhea, abdominal cramping.

Generic	**Trade**
Folic Acid	Folate
	Folvite

Classification:
Vitamin, water soluble

Pregnancy Category A

Comments
Available: PO, IM , IV, SC
Used to treat: Megaloblastic anemia. Given during pregnancy to enhance normal fetal growth and development. Stimulates production of RBCs, WBCs, and platelets.
Implications: Monitor folic acid levels, along with hemoglobin, hematocrit, and reticulocyte count. Crosses the placenta and is found in breast milk. Administer cautiously in undiagnosed anemias. Encourage foods high in folic acid: green leafy vegetables, fruits, organ meats.
Common side effects:
Rash, deep yellow urine

Generic	**Trade**
Hydroxyzine	Vistaril
	Atarax
Classification:	Vistaject-25
Sedative-hypnotic	Vistaject-50
antihistamine	

Pregnancy Category C

Comments
Available: PO, IM
Used to treat: Nausea and vomiting, anxiety, severe itching related to allergies and to enhance analyze effect of narcotic. Also used for preoperative sedation.
Implications: Contraindicated in early pregnancy but is used during labor. Safety during lactation unknown. Provide for safety as sedation occurs. Tablets can be crushed. Administer with food, very irritating to tissue, give deep, Z-tract if administered IM. Do not use deltoid muscle. Rotate sites if multiple injections given.
Common side effects
Drowsiness, dry mouth, painful IM injection, abscess may occur if not given deep IM.

Generic	**Trade**
Iron Dextran	Dextraron
	Imferon
Classification:	Irodex
Anti-anemic,	Nor-Feran10B
iron supplement	

Pregnancy Category C

Comments
Available: IM, IV
Used to treat: Iron-deficiency anemia
Implications: Give Z-track deep IM into buttocks (never the arm) with a 2-3 inch, 19 or 20 gauge needle. Infuse slowly IV (100 mg over 1-6 hours) or hypotension may occur. Crosses the placenta and is found in breast milk. Do not give oral iron preparations at the same time as parenteral administration. Absorption when taken with Vitamin C for empty stomach: absorption with tea or milk; can be taken at bedtime or with meal to aid gastric irritation.
Common side effects:
Constipation, diarrhea

Generic
Methylergonovine

Classification:
Oxytocic

Trade
Methergine
Methyler-
gobasine

Pregnancy Category C

Comments
Available: PO, IM, IV
Used to treat: Or prevent hemorrhage caused by uterine atony; postpartum or post abortion.
Monitor: Blood pressure, pulse, uterine contractions; notify physician if contractions do not occur.
Implications: Do not administer to induce labor. Use with extreme caution during third stages of labor. Found in breast milk, but in small amounts.
Common side effects:
Nausea, vomiting, cramping, hypotension, allergic reactions, signs of ergotism: cold extremities, numbness, chest pain, headache, malaise, nausea and vomiting.

Generic
Metronidazole

Classification:
Trichomonacide
Amebicide

Pregnancy Category B

Comments
Available: PO, IV, Topical
Used to treat: Gynecologic infections, especially
trichomoniasis, intra-abdominal infections, bone and joint
infections (anaerobic infections).
Implications: Monitor closely for super infection.
Contraindicated in first trimester. Crosses placenta and is found
in breast milk.
Common side effects:
Headache, dizziness, nausea and vomiting, abdominal pain,
anorexia, diarrhea, superinfection.

Generic
Oxymorphone

Trade
Numorphan

Classification:
Narcotic
analgesic-agonist
Schedule II

Pregnancy Category B

Comments
Available as: SC, IM, IV Rectal
Used to treat: Moderate to Severe pain, supplement to anesthesia.
Implications: Chronic use in pregnancy and lactation is contraindicated. Crosses the placenta and is found in breast milk, can lead to physical and psychological dependence.
Common side effects:
Sedation, confusion, constipation, respiratory depression.

Generic	**Trade**
Oxytocin	Pitocin
	Syntocinon

Classification
Hormone
Oxytocic

Pregnancy Category B

Comments
Available: IV,Intranasal
Used to facilitate: Uterine contractions and induction of labor, control postpartal bleeding, as nasal preparation to promote the let down of milk in the lactating woman.
Implications: Monitor blood pressure. Use very cautiously in first and second stages of labor, anticipated CS section, and intranasal any time during pregnancy. Assess fetal heart rate, presentation, and gestational age before administration. Monitor uterine contractions and FHR and maternal vital signs throughout administration. For induction of labor administer only as an IV piggyback preferably using an intravenous pump.
Common side effects:
Hypotension, painful contractions, signs of water intoxications: headache, confusion, restlessness, anuria.
Fetus: Intracranial bleed, hypoxia, dysrhythmias

Generic
Penicillin
G. Benzathine

Classification:
Anti-infective

Trade
Bicillin
Bicillin C-R
L-A
Permapen

Pregnancy Category B

Comments
Available: PO, IM
Used to treat: Wide range of infections, including,
pneumococcal pneumonia, streptococcal pharyngitis, syphilis.
Implications: Watch for allergic reaction obtain C & S
cultures before initiating therapy. Give on empty stomach 1 hr
before or 2 hrs. after meals. Use cautiously in pregnancy and
lactation. Avoid giving with juice or carbonated drinks. After
IM administration, massage well. Crosses the placenta and is
found in breast milk.
Common side effects:
Nausea, vomiting, diarrhea, rash, pain IM site.
Signs of anaphylaxis: Rash, itching, wheezing, laryngeal edema.

Generic
Penicillin
Potassium

Trade
Crystapen
Megacillin
P-50
Nora-Pen G
Pfizerpen
Pfizerpen G

‾
Classification:
Anti-infective

Pregnancy Category B

Comments
Available: PO, IM, IV
Used to treat: Broad spectrum of infections including
pneumococcal pneumonia, streptococcal pharyngitis, syphilis,
gonorrhea, Lyme's disease.
Implications: Monitor for allergic reaction. Do not give with
food, fruit juice or carbonated drinks: obtain C & S cultures
before initiating therapy, watch for superinfection. Use
cautiously in pregnancy and lactation. Crosses the placenta
and is found in breast milk.
Common side effects:
Nausea and vomiting, diarrhea, abdominal distress, rash, pain
at IM site, phlebitis at IV site, allergic reactions.

Generic	**Trade**	
Promethazine	Anergan 25,	PMS
	Anergan 50	promethazine
Classification:	(Histantil)	Pro-50
Antihistamine	K-Phen	Prometh-25
Antiemetic-	Mallergan	Prometh-50
Sedative/Hypnotic	Pentazine	promethergan
	Phenameth	Prorex-25
	Phenazine 25,	Prorex-50
Pregnancy	Phenazine 50	prothazine
Category C	Phencen 50	plain,
	Phenergan	V-Gan 25
	Phenergan Fortis	V-Gan 50
	Phenergan Plain	
	Phenoject 50	

Comments
Available: PO, IM, IV, Rectal
Used to treat: and prevent
Nausea and vomiting Used as an or adjunct to analgesia for labor
Implications: Monitor level of sedation. May cause EPS usually takes effect within 20 minutes. Administer with food or milk to decrease GI irritation. Used safely during labor, but avoid prolonged use during pregnancy. Use cautiously in lactation. crosses the placenta
Common side effects: Sedation, dizziness, hypotension, hypertension, dry mouth, constipation, Signs of EPS: restlessness, twitching, tremors, drooling.

Generic	**Trade**
Rh (D) Immune	RhoGAM
Globulin	RhoGAM
Standard Dose	MICRhoGAM, Mini-
Rh (D) Globulin	Gamulin Rh
MICRODOSE	

Classification:
*Serum immune
globulin*

Pregnancy Category C

Comments
Available: IM
Used to treat: Rh negative woman who has delivered an Rh positive infant, had a miscarriage or abortion, experienced amniocentesis.

Prevents the production of antibodies in Rh negative patients and prevents erythroblastosis fetalis (hemolytic disease) in the newborn in future pregnancies.

Implications: Give in deltoid. Do not give IV. Must be administered within 72 hours of exposure to Rh positive blood and prophylactics at 28 weeks to prevent maternal sensitization. Type and crossmatch both the blood of the mother and the newborn to determine need for RhoGAM. Mother must be negative and infant must be positive.

Common side effects:
Fever, painful Im injection.

Generic	**Trade**
Phytonadione	AquaMEPHYTON
	Vitamin K

Classification
Vitamin
Fat   soluble

Pregnancy
Category C

Comments
Available: SC, IM
Used to prevent: Hemorrhagic disease of the newborn.
Implication: Carefully monitor for occult bleeding or obvious
bleed 2nd or 3rd day of life. Administer : prophylactically 1
after birth; protect drug from light. Parenteral route, not IV, is
preferred.
Common side effects:
Rash, pain at injection site, bleeding, allergic reaction.

MEDICATIONS USED IN COMPLICATIONS OF CHILDBEARING

Generic	**Trade**
Digitalis glycoside	Lanoxin
Digoxin	Lanoxicaps

Classification
Cardiac glycoside
Inotropic agent
Anti-arrhythmic

Pregnancy Category C

Comments
Available: Caps, Tabs, Elix, inj
Used to treat: Congestive heart failure.
Increases cardiac output and decreases heart rate.
Implications: Use with caution in pregnancy and lactation (has been used without adverse effects to fetus). Do not give if heart rate is below 60. Do not give with antacids. Crosses placenta and is found in breast milk.
Common side effects:
Fatigue, bradycardia, nausea, vomiting, anorexia

Generic
Methyldopa (Oral)[*]

Trade
Aldomet
Dopamet
Novomedopa

Generic
Methyldopate[*]
Intravenous

Trade
Aldomet

Classification
Antihypertensive

Pregnancy Category C

Comments
Available: Tabs, Oral susp, inj
Used to treat: High blood pressure by decreasing peripheral resistance
Implications: Monitor blood pressure and pulse closely.
Use cautiously in pregnancy and lactation (it has been used safely in pregnancy)
Crosses placenta and is found in small amounts in breast milk.
Common side effects: Sedation, edema, nasal stuffiness, hypotension, depression, bradycardia, diarrhea.

*Note this drug has 2 generic names and two sets of trade names

Generic:
Betamethasone

Classification:
*Corticosteroid
synthetic*

Trade
Betnelan
Celestone/Alphatrex
Betamethasone
Dipropionate
Diprosone
Maxivate

Teladar/Diprolene
Diprolene
AT/Betamethasone
Sodium Phosphate
Sodium Phosphate
Celestone Phosphate
Cel-V-Jec,
Selestoject

*Pregnancy
Category C*

Comments
Used to treat:
Available: PO,IM,IV
Used to prevent prenatal respiratory distress syndrome
Implications:
Monitor potassium, blood sugar, urine glucose on long-term
therapy; hypokalemi a, hyperglycemia
Common side effects:
Acne, poor wound healing, ecchymosis, bruising, depression,
flushing, sweating, hypertension, diarrhea, nausea, abdominal
distention, increased appetite

Generic: **Trade**
Cefaclor   Ceclor

Classification:
Antibiotic

Pregnancy Category B

Comments
Available: Caps 250, 500 mg; oral susp. 125, 250 mg/5 ml
Used to treat:
Gram-negative bacilli, H. influenzae, E. coli, P. mirabilis,
Klebsiella, gram-positive organisms: S. Pneumoniae, S.
Pyogenes, S. aureus; upper and lower respiratory tract,
urinary tract, skin infections, otitis media.
Implications:
Assess for sensitivity to penicillins and other cephalosporins,
Nephrotoxicity; increased BUN creatinine, I and O, Blood
studies, electrolytes bowel pattern qd.
Common side effects:
Diarrhea, anorexia
Antidote: Calcium Gluconate

Generic: **Trade**
Cefadroxil   Cefadroxil
                               Duricef
Classification: Ultracef
Antibiotic

Pregnancy Category B

Comments
Available: Caps 300 mg; tabs 1g; oral susp., 125, 250,
500mg/5ml
Used to treat: Gram negative bacilli: E. coli, P. mirabilis,
Klebsiella (UTI only); gram positive organisms: S.
pneumoniae, S. pyogenes, S. aureus; upper, lower respiratory
tract, urinary tract, skin infections, otitis media, tonsillitis;
particularly for UTI
Implications: Assess sensitivity to penicillin; other
cephalosporins; nephrotoxicity; increased BUN; I and O
daily; Blood studies, electrolytes, bowel pattern qd.
Common side effects:
Diarrhea, anorexia

Drugs from the cephalosporins have many of the same side effects and uses.
The drug is chosen based on strain of infection, and cost.

Generic:
Diazepam

Classification:
Antianxiety

Pregnancy Category D

Trade
Diazepam
Diazepam Intensol
D-Tran
Valium
Val Release
Vasepam 2
Zetran

Comments:
Available: Tabs 2, 5, 10 mg; caps ext rel 15 mg, IM/ IV
inj
Used to treat: Anxiety; seizures
Implications: Assess blood pressure; pulse, blood studies,
hepatic studies
Common side effects: Dizziness, drowsiness, orthostatic
hypotension, blurred vision

Generic: **Trade**
Folic acid(Vitamin B9)   Apofolic
                                       Folvite,
Classification: Novofolacid*
*Vitamin B Complex
group*

Pregnancy Category A

Comments:
Available: Tabs 0.1, 0.4, 0.8, 1 mg; inj SC, IM, IV 5, 10
mg/ml
Used to treat: Megaloblastic or macrocytic anemia resulting
from folic acid deficiency; liver disease, alcoholism,
hemolysis, intestinal obstruction, pregnancy
Implications: Assess Hgb, Hct and reticulocyte count
Folate levels: 6-15 µml
Common side effects: None known

Generic:	**Trade**
Furosemide	Fumide
	Furomide
Classification:	M.D . Furosemide
Loop diuretic	Lasix
	Luramide

Pregnancy Category C

Comments
Available: Tabs 20, 40, 80 mg; oral sol 10 mg/ml, inj. IM, IV 10 mg/ml

Used to treat: Pulmonary edema, edema in CHF, liver disease, nephrotic syndrome, ascites, hypertension

Implications: Assess hearing, weight loss, I and O daily for fluid loss; rate depth, rhythm of respirations, effect of exertion, blood pressure lying, standing, postural hypotension, electrolytes, potassium, sodium, chloride glucose in urine of diabetic patient

Common side effects:
Polyuria, hypokalemia, hypochloremic alkalosis, hypomagnesemia, hyperuricemia, hypocalcemia, nausea

Generic:
Gentamicin

Classification
Antibiotic

Pregnancy
Category C

Trade

Alcomin
Apogen
Cidomycin
Garamycin
Garamycin
Intrathecal
Pediatric
Gentamicin
Sulfate

Garamycin IV
Piggyback
Garamycin
Pediatric
Gentamicin
Sulfate
Gentamicin
Sulfate IV
Piggyback
Jenamicin

Comments
Available: Inj, IM IV
Used to treat: Urinary tract infections, bone, skin, soft tissues
Implications: Assess weight before treatment, dosage calculation is based on weight; I&O ratio, daily urinalysis, VS during infusion; IV site for thrombophlebitis including pain, redness, swelling; serum peak, urine Ph if used for urinary tract infections.
Common side effects:
Nausea, vomiting, anorexia, rash

Generic:
Hydralazine

Classification:
Antihypertensive
direct-acting peripheral
vasodilator

Trade
Alazine
Apresoline
Hydralazine HCl

Pregnancy CategoryC

Comments
Available: PO,IV,IM
Used to treat: Essential hypertension
Implications: Assess B/P q 5min x 2hr, q 1h x 2h,4h.
Monitor pulse, jugular venous distention, electrolytes, blood
studies, potassium, sodium, chloride
Common side effects:
Lupuslike symptoms, palpitations, reflex tachycardia, angina,
shock, headache, tremors, dizziness, anxiety, nausea,
vomiting, anorexia, diarrhea

Generic:
Magnesium sulfate

Classification:
Anticonvulsant

Pregnancy Category C

Comments:
Available: Inj., IV, IM, 10%, 50%, 12.5%, 25%, granules
Used to treat: Hypomagnesemic seizures, control of
seizures in pregnancy-induced hypertension, seizures in acute
nephritis
Implications: Assess VS q 15 min after IV dose; do not
exceed 150 mg/min; monitor cardiac function; magnesium
levels; timing of contractions, determine intensity; fetal heart
rate; reactivity may decrease with this drug if using during
labor
Common side effects:
Sweating, depressed deep tendon reflexes, flushing,
hypotension

Generic:	**Trade**
Nifedipine	Adalat
	Nifedipine
Classification:	Procardia
Calcium - channel blocker	Procardia XL

Pregnancy Category C

Comments

Available: Caps 10, 20 mg, Tabs sus rel 30, 60, 90 mg

Used to treat: Chronic stable angina pectoris, vasospastic angina, hypertension (sustained release only)

Implications: Monitor cardiac status: blood pressure, pulse, respiration, ECG

Common side effects:

Dysrhythmia, edema, nausea, rash, headache, fatigue, drowsiness

Generic:
Penicillin G procaine

Classification:
Broad spectrum, long-acting antibiotic

Trade
Crysticillin A.S.,
Duracillin A.S.,
Wycillin
Pfizerpen-AS

Pregnancy Category B

Comments
Available: Inj., IM 300,000, 500,000, 600,000 U/ml,
600,000/1.2 ml, 1,200,000 U/dose, 2,000,000 U/dose
Used to treat: Gonorrhea, urinary tract infections
*Implications:*Assess I and O; monitor for hematuria,
oliguria;toxicity may occur in patient with compromised
renal system.
Common side effects:
Nausea, vomiting, diarrhea, vaginitis, moniliasis

Generic:
Penicillin G Sodium

Trade
Crystapen
Pfizerpan

Classification:
Broad spectrum antibiotic

Pregnancy Category B

Comments
Available: Inj. IM, IV 1 million, .5 million, 20 million U
Used to treat: Gonorrhea, urinary tract infections
Implications: Monitor I and O, hematuria, oliguria; monitor
patients with poor renal system; drug is excreted slowly in
these patients with poor renal systems. Assess liver studies,
blood studies, renal studies, C and S before drug therapy
Common side effects:
Nausea, vomiting, diarrhea

Generic	**Trade**
Propylthiouracil (PTU)	Propyl-Thyracil*
	Propylthiouracil

Classification:
Thyroid hormone antagonist

Pregnancy Category D

Comments
Available: Tabs, 50 mg
Used to treat: Hyperthyroidism, weight gain
Implications: Monitor for hypersensitivity: rash, enlarged cervical nodes; hypoprothrombinemia, bone marrow depression
Common side effects:
Rash, urticaria, pruritus, alopecia, hyperpigmentation, drowsiness, headache, vertigo, fever, nausea, diarrhea, vomiting

Generic	Trade
Propranolol HCl	Inderal
	Inderal LA
Classification:	Inderal 10
B-Adrenergic blocker	Inderal 20
	Inderal 40
	Inderal 60
Pregnancy Category C	Inderal 80
	Ipran
	Propranolol HCl
	Propranolol Intensol

Comments

Available: Caps, tabs, inj., Conc oral, sol 80mg/ml, ext red
cap 60mg

Used to treat: Chronic stable angina pectoris, hypertension,
supraventricular dysrhythmias, antidote in tocalytic therapy
of (ritodrine or terbutaline).

Implications: Monitor blood pressure, pulse, respirations
during beginning therapy. Report weight of five pounds,
monitor I and O ratio CrCl if kidney damage diagnosed,
ECG if using antidysrhythmic

Common side effects: Bronchospasm, hypotension,
bradycardia

Generic
Insulin, regular

Classification:
Exogenous unmodified insulin
Pregnancy Category B

Trade
Beef Regular
Iletin II
Humulin BA
Humuli n R
Novolin R
Pork Regular
Iletin II
Regular purified Pork
Novolin R Pen Fill
Velosulin

Comments
Available: IV/IM/SC/inj. U40, U100/ml
Used to treat: Adult onset diabetes, juvenile diabetes, ketoacidosis, type I, II, NIDDM, IDDM, Gestational Diabetes, hyperkalemia
Implications: Assess for fasting blood glucose, 2 hr PP (60-100mg/dl normal fasting level) (70-130 mg/dl normal 2hr level) Urine ketones during illness; insulin requirements increase during times of stress, illness, gestation progression in second & third trimesters
Common side effects:
Hypoglycemia

Generic
Insulin
Isophane Suspension NPH
Classification:
Exogenous unmodified
insulin

Pregnancy Category B

Trade
Beef NPH
Iletin II
Humulin N
Insulated NPH
NPH Iletin I
Pork NPA
Iletin II
NPH Insulin
NPH purified Pork

Comments
Available: SC 40, 100U/ml
Used to treat: Ketoacidosis, type I (IDDM), type II
(NIDDM) diabetes mellitus, Gestational Diabetes
hyperkalemia
Implications: Assess fasting blood glucose, 2 hr PP (80-
150 mg/dl. Normal fasting level) (70-130 mg/dl normal 2 hr
level) Urine ketones during times of illness, insulin
requirements may increase during times of stress, illness,
gestation progression in second & third trimesters
Common side effects:
Hypoglycemia

Generic	**Trade**
Levothyroxine sodium	Levothroid
	Levothyroxine Sodium
Classification:	Levoxine,
Thyroid hormone	Synthroid

Pregnancy Category A

Comments
Available: Inj., IV 200, 500 ng/vial; tabs 0.025, 0.05, 0.075, 0.088, 0.1, 0.112, 0.125, 0.15, 0.175, 0.2, 0.3 mg
Used to treat: Hypothyroidism, thyroid hormone replacement
Implications: Assess Blood pressure before each dose; I & O ratio, Weight qd; pro-time may necessitate decreased anti-coagulant
Common side effects: Anxiety, insomnia, tremors, tachycardia, palpitations, angina, dysrhythmias

Generic   **Trade**
Ritodrine HCl   Yutopar

Classification:
Tocolytic
uterine relaxant

Comments:
Available: Tabs 10 mg; inj. 10 mg/ml, 15 mg/ml
Used to treat: Pre-term labor
Implications: Assess for maternal, fetal heart tones during
infusion; intensity length of uterine contractions; fluid intake
to prevent fluid overload; monitor blood glucose in diabetics
Common side effects: Rash, hyperventilation, headache,
restlessness, anxiety, nervousness, sweating, nausea,
vomiting, anorexia, constipation

Generic:
Sodium bicarbonate

Classification:
Alkalinizer
Pregnancy category C

Comments
Available as: Tabs 325, 520, 650 mg; powd; inj. 40%,
4.2%, 5%, 7.5%, 8.4%
Used to treat: Metabolic acidosis, cardiac arrest,
alkanization (systemic/urinary), antacid
Implications: Monitor respiratory rate and pulse rate,
rhythm, depth, lung sounds,; Assess for edema, I and O,
urine pH; monitor electrolytes, blood pH, Pos, HCO3 during
treatment, ABGs during emergency situations
Common side effects:
Twitching, hyperreflexia, belching, distention, alkalosis

Generic
Sulfadiazine

Classification:
Antibiotic

Pregnancy Category C

Comments
Available: Tabs 500 mg
Used to treat: Urinary tract infections
Implications: I and O ratio; color, character, pH of urine.
Monitor for desired output of 800 ml less than intake
Common side effects:
Nausea, vomiting, abdominal pain

Generic: **Trade**
Sulfamethizole   Sulfasol
                      Thiosulfil

Classification:
Antibiotic

Pregnancy Category
C

Comments
Available: Tabs 250, 500 mg
Used to treat: Urinary tract infections
Implications: Assess I & O, note color, character of urine;
assess for desired output of 800 ml less than intake
Common side effects:
Nausea, vomiting, abdominal pain

Generic
Terbutaline sulfate

Classification:
Selective B2-agonist

Trade
Brethaire,
Brethine
Bricanyl

Pregnancy Category B

Comments
Available: Tabs 2.5, 5mg; aerosol 0.2mg/actuation
Used to treat: Bronchospasm, premature labor (in special
Implications: Assess respiratory function, vital capacity,
forced expiratory volume ABG's, B/P, pulse
Common side effects:
Tremors, anxiety

Generic	**Trade**
Heparin	Calcilean Calciparine
	Heparin
Classification:	Heparin Sodium
	Sodium Chloride
Anticoagulant	Heparin Lock Flush
	Heparin Sodium
Pregnancy category C	Hep-Lock
	Liquaemin Sodium

Comments
Available: IV, inj.
Used to treat: Deep vein thrombosis, pulmonary emboli, myocardial infarction, open heart surgery, disseminated intravascular clotting syndrome, atrial fibrillation, as an anticoagulant in transfusion and dialysis procedures
Implications: Assess blood studies, PTT, APTT, ACT
Monitor blood pressure for increasing signs of hypertension
Common side effects:
Diarrhea, rash, fever

Toxic Chemical Agents

- Alcohol
- Chemotherapeutic agents
- Chloroquine
- Carbon monoxide
- Coumarins
- Lead
- LSD
- Methamphetamine
- Salicylates
- Tetracycline

- Arsenic
- Barbiturates
- Cigarette smoking
- Cocaine
- Heroine
- Lithium carbonate
- Mercury
- Radiation
- Streptomycin
- Thalidomide

Nursing Interventions Used in Obstetric Emergencies

Prenatal Hemorrhage

- Whole blood
- Packed RBCs

Postpartal Hemorrhage

- Fresh Frozen Plasma with Platelets
- Methergine (methylergonovine)

- Oxytocin
- Prostaglandin F2a

- Blood

Severe PIH and Eclampsia

- Magnesium sulfate
- Phenobarbital sodium
- Valium (diazepam)

NURSING CARE
PLANNING

NURSING CARE PLANNING

THE NURSING PROCESS

The term "Nursing Process" was first used in 1955 and since then has become the hallmark of quality nursing care. The nursing process is a systematic, cyclic process which evolves into five steps that emphasize individualized care. Nurses are charged with the accountability of implementing the nursing process.

The five steps of the nursing process are assessment, nursing diagnosis, planning or outcome criteria, intervention, and evaluation. Each part of the process has its specific criteria for nursing action:

1. Assessing the patient's condition.
2. Identifying and stating the problem with a nursing diagnosis.
3. Planning priorities of care with specific outcome criteria.
4. Intervening to effectively implement that plan.
5. Evaluating the patient's response and outcome based upon outcome criteria.

The nursing process begins with the interview and history. When the assessment is complete, a nursing diagnosis is made, patient goals are set, outcome criteria for evaluation is determined and nursing interventions are ordered. Once this cycle is completed, reassessment is necessary. The nurse explores why and how the plan of care did or did not work.

Assessment and nursing diagnoses are the foundation of
the nursing process and the nursing care plan. In order to
effectively utilize nursing diagnoses, it is important to
understand the three components of a nursing diagnosis,
all of which must be documented. They are:

- Statement of the problem. Identifying conditions
  from the NANDA list of nursing diagnoses that address independent nursing care.
- Etiology of the problem: Identifying the probable
  cause of a patient's problem or potential problem.

Defining characteristics of the problem. Selecting the
specific objective and subjective data gathered during the
assessment that relate to this particular problem. Each
component of the nursing process along with a specific
design resulting in specific nursing actions is summarized
in the following table.

THE NURSING PROCESS IN ACTION

THE PROCESS

Assessment

THE DESIGN

- Collect, verify and organize the data. Recognize
  problems and potential problems. Ask the question: "What's going on with this patient in this
  situation?"

THE ACTION

Interview

- Patient history
- Physical exam
- Lab data

- Physician's history
- Systems assessment

THE PROCESS

Nursing diagnosis

• Specifically identify and label problems and potential problems. Ask the question, "What is the problem and the potential problem in this situation?"

THE ACTION

Analyze data.

• Derive nursing diagnosis from the NANDA list. Establish the priority of problems identified.

THE PROCESS

Planning/Outcome Criteria

• Plan priorities of care that are realistic for that individual. Patient-oriented goals, called outcome criteria, must be measurable and specific. These criteria are the basis upon which evaluation will be made. Ask the question, "What can the patient accomplish in this situation?"

THE ACTION

• Determine what the patient is able to achieve and ask the patient for input in the plan of care. Give the patient as much control as possible. Delegate action and decide upon the focus of decision.

THE PROCESS

Intervention

• What will the nurse do to help the patient accomplish care plan goals? Determine what the dependent interventions and independent interventions will be. Ask the question, "What can I do to help the patient in this situation?"

THE ACTION

- Perform nursing interventions. Begin reassessing what works and what does not. Be sure to intervene based on scientific rationales whether they are actually written on the care plan or not.

THE PROCESS

Evaluation

- Determine to what extent goals have been achieved. Assess patient response. Evaluate progress based upon outcome criteria. Ask the question, "Is the patient better or worse? Why?"

THE ACTION

- Compare patient response to outcome criteria. Analyze why the patient responded the way he did. Reassess. Update care plan. Ask the question, "What do we do now?"

GUIDELINES FOR THERAPEUTIC COMMUNICATION IN A HELPING RELATIONSHIP

- ❖ Be congruent in what you are saying and what your body language is conveying.

- ❖ Use clear, concise words that are adapted to the individual's intelligence and experience.

- ❖ Do not say, "I understand." Nonverbally or verbally say, "I care about you."

- ❖ Use appropriate silence to give the patient time to organize his thoughts.

- ❖ Let the patient set the pace of the exchange—do not hurry him.

- ❖ Accept the patient as he is. The nursing profession espouses empathy without judgment.

- ❖ Offer a collaborative relationship in which you are willing to work with the patient in resolving problems but not to resolve these problems for him.

- ❖ Use open-ended questions to encourage expression of feelings and ideas.

- ❖ Explore ideas completely. Do not drop a subject that the patient has brought up without some resolution.

- ❖ Clarify statements and relationships when necessary. Do not try to read the patient's mind.

- ❖ Give positive feedback every chance you get. Praise the patient for communication and attempts at problem-solving.

- ❖ Encourage expression of feelings.

- ❖ Paraphrase statements and feelings to facilitate further talking.

- ❖ Translate feelings into words so that hidden meanings can be discovered.

- ❖ Focus on reality, especially if the patient misinterprets the facts or if he is misrepresenting the truth.

- ❖ Offer teaching and information, but avoid giving advice.

- ❖ Search for mutual, intuitive understanding. Encourage the patient to ask for clarification if he does not understand what is being said. Do not use slang or phrases that can be misunderstood.

❖ Encourage an appropriate plan of action, such as problem-solving or self-care.

❖ Summarize at the end of the conversation to focus on the important points of the communication and validate the patient's understanding.

❖ Remember, the more personal and intense a feeling or thought is, the more difficult it is to communicate. Give the patient the time and the security to express his deepest feelings. The key word is *listen*.

BARRIERS TO THERAPEUTIC COMMUNICATION

Therapeutic communication techniques are valuable. However, the attitude of caring is the foundation of therapeutic transaction. The nurse should be aware of actions that often block communication.

- Using words that the patient does not understand or inappropriate cliches.
- Inferring to the patient that you are in a hurry or preoccupied with other tasks.
- Showing anger or anxiety, especially when those feelings provoke an argument with the patient.
- Incorrectly interpreting what the patient expresses.
- Offering counseling when the timing is wrong or when the patient is not ready to hear what is being communicated.
- Giving false reassurance and discounting the patient's feelings.

- Expressing opinions and giving advice, especially when these feelings provoke an argument with the patient.
- Persistently asking probing questions that make the patient uncomfortable.
- Being insincere. (Patients pick this up very quickly.)
- Interrupting while the patient is talking.

DOCUMENTATION—THE VITAL LINK TO COMMUNICATION

The purpose of charting is to communicate the care given to the patient. Documentation of nursing care must be as complete and congruent as the care itself. Documentation is the best way for a nurse to provide accountability in situations where she is responsible for patient care. The battle cry on the documentation front has become: "If it is not charted, it is not done."

WHAT TO CHART

The Head-to-Toe Systems Assessment. Get a general impression of what is going on with the patient; then focus on particular problems. Carefully assess the situation by asking yourself:

What do I see?_____

What do I hear?_____

What do I think? _____

What will I do? _____

What should I do?_____

What has already been done?_____

How is the patient responding? _____

The nursing process must be charted each shift by recording a nursing physical assessment, nursing diagnoses based on problems and potential problems, goals of patient care, nursing interventions and an evaluation of the patient's progress.

- Any change in conditions, especially if the patient's condition is deteriorating.
- Be as specific as possible, using descriptive details rather than conveying a judgmental tone.
- Include patient response to any treatment or medication.
- Describe patient's understanding of any health teaching.
- Show continuity of care, especially with treatments that require frequent monitoring, such as IV therapy.
- Patient's medical diagnosis and treatments should be noted at least once each shift.
- Indicate all contacts with the physician, including details and direct quotes when pertinent.
- Chart exact times of patient activities, treatments or procedures.
- Chart patient care at least every two hours.
- Correlate documentation regarding the nursing care plan, physician's orders and treatment plan.

HOW TO CHART

- Always chart in the correct color of ink.
- Write legibly using accurate and concise medical terminology.
- Spell correctly.
- Addressograph and date must be on each page.
- Do not skip lines.

- Do not write between the lines.
- Do not skip times—chart in a time sequence.
- Chart at least every two hours.
- Do not chart in advance of nursing care administered.
- Close entries with name and title.
- Designate late entries as LATE ENTRY with the time.
- Make one line through an error, write ERROR, and sign.
- Never erase. Never use liquid coverup or erasable pens.
- If page must be recopied, draw a single diagonal line across the original and designate book "copy" and original on the appropriate page.
- Do not chart for anyone else; never let anyone else chart for you.
- Use only those abbreviations accepted by your agency.
- Use direct quotes when appropriate.
- Be objective. Do not draw conclusions or write judgments.
- Avoid such words as "good," "normal" and "appears to be."
- The more descriptive the details, the better.

PROTECTING YOURSELF LEGALLY

- There are two key elements in protecting yourself legally— documentation and respect for the patient and family. A patient who is shown respect rarely sues. However, adequate documentation is the surefire defense when a nurse is required to prove accountability.

- Complete documentation will safeguard the nurse if she becomes involved in a lawsuit. The nursing notes should reflect that the nurse practiced reasonable and prudent care under the circumstances.

- Biased feelings and judgmental thoughts should never be included in the nursing notes on the chart. Nurses should avoid the use of words such as "uncooperative" and "hostile". When these actions are recorded, they should be written as a fact using direct quotes.

- It is important that you always document that you are following the policy and procedure of the hospital. If you catheterize a patient, note that it was done by sterile technique. If you change IV tubing and the policy and procedure states that it should be done every 48 hours, make a note that this was done. Every small detail of the policy and procedure does not need to be cited. However, it should be noted that a special procedure was done according to policy and procedure.

- There are many reasons the nurse should know the policy and procedure of the hospital where she works. If there is a necessity for a particular policy, then it is important. Legally, it is of utmost importance to follow policy and procedure because if a nurse is involved in an incident, and she did not follow policy and procedure, the hospital malpractice is not obligated to defend her. When this happens, the nurse must supply her own defense. This is one reason that it is a good idea to carry private malpractice insurance.

- It is essential to document any procedure that involves the patient. If it is not charted on the medical record, legally it is not done.

MORE GUIDELINES TO PREVENT MALPRACTICE

Always exercise reasonable and prudent care under the circumstances.

- Be thoroughly knowledgeable of the hospital's policy and procedure.
- Show concern and caring about your patient.
- Show positive regard to the family. Research indicates family members are more likely to sue than the patient.
- Keep your nursing knowledge current.
- Stay knowledgeable about nursing standards of care.
- Keep current by reading nursing journals on a regular basis.
- Be selective in delegating nursing responsibilities.
- Complete charts in a timely manner.
- Always be aware of the patient's safety.
- Exercise precaution in administering medications.

PROFESSIONAL NETWORK

PROFESSIONAL NETWORK

HOW TO WRITE A RESUME

A resume should be concisely written and organized for at-a-glance reading. Employers quickly screen resumes, and they are often the basis for that important first impression. A professional resume consists of seven components.

I. The Cover Letter

- ❖ Use an appropriate business letter format.
- ❖ State the reason you are applying for the position.
- ❖ Emphasize how your qualifications meet their requirements.
- ❖ Request to schedule an interview.
- ❖ State that you have enclosed your resume.

II. Personal Data

- ❖ Name
- ❖ Address/telephone number
- ❖ Professional license number
- ❖ Social security number
- ❖ Sex
- ❖ Age
- ❖ Race

III. Job Objectives
- ❖ Type of position you are seeking
- ❖ How your abilities and skills qualify you for this position.

IV. Educational Background
- ❖ Where and when you went to school
- ❖ Degrees earned
- ❖ Continuing education courses taken

V. Work Experience
- ❖ Place and dates of employment, beginning with present. Include volunteer work when applicable.
- ❖ Concisely emphasize major work responsibilities.

VI. Extracurricular Activities
- ❖ Personal development
- ❖ Hobbies
- ❖ Professional organizations

VII. References
Names and addresses of three persons. Include one personal and two professional references. Avoid the names of relatives.

GUIDELINES TO A SUCCESSFUL JOB INTERVIEW

What will the interviewer ask? The following are broad statements that will cover inquiries during the interview.

- Tell about yourself. Briefly and concisely outline your strengths. Concentrate on your professional, not personal, accomplishments.

- Tell about your qualifications for the job.

- List your strongest and most recent qualifications. Tell why you want the job. Know something about the employer. Be able to say something positive about the company. Avoid using money as a reason.

- Never be critical about past employers, especially if you are changing jobs. Avoid negative comments throughout the interview.

- Tell about your ambitions. Mention that you look forward to new challenges and responsibilities.

- Mention strengths in regard to your new position.

- Mention weaknesses or problems that have been good experiences for you.

- Tell about your salary requirements. Give a range based on an annual wage. De-emphasize money as your motivation for wanting the job.

BOARDS OF NURSING BY STATE

The following is a list of the state boards of nursing and continuing education requirements for each state

State	Board of Nursing	CE Requirements
Alabama	Board of Nursing RSA Plaza, Suite 250 770 Washington Avenue Montgomery, AL 36130 (205) 242-4060	24 hours every 2 years beginning in 1993
Alaska	Board of Nursing 3601 C. Street, Suite 722 Anchorage, AK 99503 (907) 561-2878	30 contact hours in 2 years for nurse practitioners
Arizona	Board of Nursing 2001 W. Camelback #350 Phoenix, AZ 85015 602-271-0592	None
Arkansas	State Board of Nursing 1123 South University Suite 800 Little Rock, AR 72204 (501) 686-2700	None
California	Board of Nursing Box 944210 Sacramento, CA 94244-2100 (916) 322-3350	30 contact hours every 2 years

Colorado	Board of Nursing 1560 Broadway Suite 670 Denver, CO 80202 (303) 894-2430	20 contact hours every 2 years
Connecticut	Board of Nursing 150 Washington Hartford, CT 06106 (203) 566-1041	None
Delaware	Board of Nursing Margaret O' Neil Building Box 1041 Dover, DE 19903 (302) 739-4522	30 contact hours every 2 years
District of Columbia	Nurses Examining Board 614 H Street, N.W. Room 112 Washington, D.C. 20001 (202) 727-7823	None
Florida	Board of Nursing 111 East Coastline Drive Suite 516 Jacksonville, FL 32202 (904) 359-6341	24 contact hours every 2 years
Georgia	Board of Nursing 166 Pryor Street, S.W. Suite 400 Atlanta, GA 30303 (404) 656-3943	None

Hawaii	Board of Nursing Box 3469 Honolulu, HI 96801 (808) 548-7471	None
Idaho	Board of Nursing 280 North 8th Street Suite 210 Boise, ID 83720 (208) 334-3110	Nurse prac- titioners 60 contact hours every 2 years
Illinois	Department of Professional Regulation 320 West Washington Street Third Floor Springfield, IL 62786 (217) 782-0458	None
Indiana	Board of Nurses Registration One American Square Suite 1020 Indianapolis, IN 46282 (317) 232-2960	None
Iowa	Board of Nursing 1223 E. Court Avenue Des Moines, IA 50319 (515) 281-3255	45 contact hours every 3 years

Kansas	Board of Nursing P.O. Box 1098 503 Kansas Avenue Suite 330 Topeka, KS 66601 (913) 296-4929	30 contact hours every 2 years
Kentucky	Board of Nursing 4010 DuPont Circle, Suite 430 Louisville, KY 40207 (502) 897-5143	30 contact hours every 2 years, in- cluding 2 hours of HIV/AIDS education
Lousiana	Board of Nursing 150 Baronne Street, Room 912 New Orleans, LA 70112 (504) 568-5464	30 contact hours every 2 years, or 20 hours plus 320 hours active practice
Maine	Board of Nursing 158 State House Station Augusta, ME 04333 (207) 289-5324	None
Maryland	Board of Nursing 201 West Preston Street Baltimore, MD 21201 (301) 383-2084	None

Massachusetts	Board of Registration in Nursing Leverett Saltonstall Bldg. Government C enter 100 Cambridge Street Boston, MA 02202 (617) 727-9961	15 contact hours every 2 years
Michigan	Board of Nursing Box 30018 905 Southland Lansing, MI 48909 (517) 373-1600	None
Minnesota	Board of Nursing 2700 University Avenue West # 108 Saint Paul, MN 55114 (612) 642-0575	30 contact hours every 2 years
Mississippi	Board of Nursing 239 N. Lamar Number 401 Jackson, MS 39201 (601) 359-6170	Nurse prac- titioners 40 hours every 2 years
Missouri	Board of Nursing Box 656 3523 N. Ten Mile Drive Jefferson City, MO 65102 (314) 751-0681	None

Montana	Board of Nursing 111 North Jackson Arcade Building, Lower Level Helena, MT 59620 (406) 444-2071	None
Nebraska	Department of Health Bureau of Examining Boards 301 Centennial Mall P.O. Box 95007 Lincoln, NE 68509 (402) 471-2115	20 contact hours and 200 hours of nursing prac- tice every 5 years, or 75 contact hours
Nevada	Board of Nursing 1281 Terminal Way Suite 116 Reno, NV 89502 (702) 786-2778	30 contact hours every 2 years
New Hampshire	Board of Nursing Education and Registration 105 Loudon Road Concord, N H 03301 (603) 271-2323	Nurse practitioners 20 hours every 2 years
New Jersey	Board of Nursing 1100 Raymond Blvd. Room 319 Newark, N J 07102 (201) 648-2490	None

New Mexico	Board of Nursing 4523 Montgomery N.E. Suite 130 Albuquerque, NM 87109 (505) 841-8340	30 hours every 2 years; 50 hours for nurse prac- titioners
New York	Board of Nursing State Education Department Cultural Education Center Albany, N Y 12230 (518) 474-3848	None
North Carolina	Board of Nursing P.O. Box 2129 Raleigh, N C 27602 (919) 782-3211	None
Ohio	Board of Nursing Education and Registration 65 South Front Street Suite 509 Columbus, OH 43215 (614) 466-3947	None
Oklahoma	Board of Nursing 2915 North Classen, Suite 524 Oklahoma City, OK 73106 (405) 525-2076	None

Oregon	Board of Nursing 10445 S.W. Canyon Rd. Beaverton, O R 97005 (503) 644-2767	Nurse prac- titioners 100 contact hours every 2 years
Pennsylvania	State Board of Nursing P.O. Box 2649 Harrisburg, PA 17105-2649 (717) 783-7142	None
Rhode Island	Board of Nursing Professional Regulation 3 Capitol Hill, Room 104 Providence, RI 02908 (401) 277-2827	None
South Carolina	Board of Nursing 220 Executive Center Drive Columbia, S C 29210-8420 (803) 731-1648	None
South Dakota	Board of Nursing 3307 South Lincoln Sioux Falls, SD 57105-5224 (605) 335-4973 Fax: (605) 335-2977	None
Tennessee	Board of Nursing 283 Plus Park Blvd Nashville, TN 37129-5407 615) 367-6232	None

Texas	Board of Nurse Examiners 1901 Burnet Road, Suite 104 Austin, Texas 78758 or (mailing address) Box 140466 Austin, TX 78714 (512) 835-4880	20 contact hours every 2 years
Utah	Department of Commerce Division of Occupational and Professional Licensing 160 East 300 South Salt Lake City, UT 84145-0805 (801) 530-6628	Must work 1200 hours
Vermont	Board of Nursing 109 State Street Montpelier, VT 05609 In Vermont: (800) 439-8683 Outside: (802) 828-2396	CEU : None Practice re- quirements: 400 hours in 2 years or 960 hours in 5 years
Virginia	Board of Nursing 1601 Rolling Hills Drive Richmond, VA 23229 (804) 662-9909	None
Washington	Board of Nursing Box 1099 Olympia, WA 98507-1099 (206) 753-3726	None

West Virginia	Board of Examiners Embleton Building, Room 309 922 Quarrier Street Charleston, WV 25301 (304) 348-3596	None
Wisconsin	Department of Regulation and Licensing Board of Nursing P.O. Box 8935 Madison, WI 53708 (608) 266-0257	None
Wyoming	State Board of Nursing 2301 Central Avenue Barrett Building, 2nd Floor Cheyenne, WY 82002 (307) 777-7601	20 hours in 2 years or practice for 500 hours in 2 years or 1600 hours in 5 years or pass RN NCLEX within last 5 years

STATE NURSE'S ASSOCIATIONS

The American Nurses Association is supported by the following 53 state organizations.

Alabama State
Nurses Association
360 North Hull Street
Montgomery, AL 36197
(205) 262-8321

Alaska Nurses
Association
237 East Third Avenue
Anchorage, AK 99501
(907) 274-0827

Arizona Nurses Association
1850 East Southern Avenue,
Suite 1
Tempe, AZ 85282
(602) 831-0404

Arkansas State Nurses
Association
117 South Cedar Street
Little Rock, AR 72205
(501) 664-5853

California Nurses Association
1855 Folsom Street, Suite 670
San Francisco, CA 94103
(415) 864-4141

Colorado Nurses
Association
5453 East Evans Place
Denver, CO 88222
(303) 575-7484

Connecticut Nurses Association
Meritech Business Park
377 Research Parkway,
Suite 2D
Meriden, Connecticut 06450
(203)238-1207

Delaware Nurses
Association
2634 CapitolTrail,
Suite A
Newark, Delaware 19711
(302) 368-2333

District of Columbia
Nurses Association
5100 Wisconsin Avenue,
N.W. Suite 306
Washington, D.C. 20016
(202) 244-2705

Georgia Nurses Association
1362 West Peachtree Street,
N. W. Atlanta, GA 30309
(404) 876-4624

Hawaii Nurses Association
677 Ala Moana Blvd,
Suite 301
Honolulu, HI 96813
(808) 531-1628 or 521-8361

Illinois Nurses Association
20 North Wacker Drive
Suite 2520
Chicago, IL 60606
(312) 236-9708

Iowa Nurses Association
100 Court Avenue, 9 LL
Des Moines, IA 50309
(515) 282-9169

Florida Nurses
Association
P.O. Box 536985
Orlando, FL 32853-
6985
(305) 896-3261

Guam Nurses Associa-
tion
P.O. Box 3134
Agana, GU 96910

Idaho Nurses Association
200 North 4th Street,
Suite 20
Boise, ID 83702-6001
(208) 345-0500

Indiana State Nurses
Association
2915 North High School
Road
Indianapolis, IN 46224
(317) 299-4575

Kansas State Nurses
Association
700 S.W. Jackson,
Suite 601
Topeka, KS 66603
(913) 233-8638

Kentucky Nurses Association
1400 South First Street
Louisville, KY 40201
(502) 637-2546

Louisiana State Nurses
Association
712 Transcontinental
Drive
Metaire, LA 70001
(504) 889-1030

Maine State Nurses Association
P.O. Box 2240
Augusta, ME 04330
(207) 622-1057

Maryland Nurses
Association
5820 Southwestern
Boulevard
Baltimore, MD 21227
(301) 242-7300

Massachusetts Nurses
Association
340 Turnpike Street
Canton, MA 02021
(617) 821-4625

Michigan Nurses
Association
120 Spartan Avenue
East Lansing, MI 48823

Minnesota Nurses Association
1295 Bandana Boulevard
North Suite 140
Saint Paul, MN
55108-5115
(612) 464-4807

Mississippi Nurses
Association
135 Bounds Street,
Suite 100
Jackson, MS 39206
(601) 982-9182

Missouri Nurses Association
206 East Dunklin Street,
Box 325
Jefferson City, MO 65101
(314) 636-4623

Montana Nurses
Association
104 Broadway,
Suite G-2
P.O. Box 5718
Helena, MT 59601
(406) 442-6710

Nebraska Nurses Association
941 "O" Street, Suite 707-711
Lincoln, NE 68508
(402) 475-3859

Nevada Nurses
Association
3660 Baker Lane,
Suite 104
Reno, NV 89509
(702) 825-3555

New Hampshire
Nurses Association
48 West Street
Concord, NH 03301
(603) 225-3783

New Jersey State
Nurses Association
320 West State Street
Trenton, N J 87018
(609) 392-4884

New Mexico Nurses
Association
303 Washington, S.E.
Albuquerque, N M 87108
(505) 268-7744

New York State
Nurses Association
2113 Western Avenue
Guilderland, NY 12084
(518) 456-5371

North Carolina
Nurses Association
Box 12025
103 Enterprise Street
Raleigh, NC 27605
(919) 821-4250

North Dakota State
Nurses Association
Green Tree Square
212 North Fourth Street
Bismark, ND 58501
(701) 223-1385

Ohio Nurses Association
4000 East Main Street
Columbus, OH 43213-2950
(614) 237-5414

Oregon Nurses Association
9600 S.W. Oak, Suite 550
Portland, OR 97223
(503) 293-0011

Rhode Island State
Nurses Association
Hall Building South
354 Blackstone Boulevard
Providence, Rhode Island 02906
(401) 421-9703

South Dakota Nurses
Association
1505 South Minnesota,
Suite # 6
Sioux Falls, South Dakota
57105
(605) 338-1401

Oklahoma Nurses
Association
6414 North Santa Fe,
Suite A
Oklahoma City, OK
73116
(405) 840-3476

Pennsylvania Nurses
Association
2578 Interstate Drive
P.O. Box 8525
Harrisburg, PA 17105-
8525
(717) 657-1222

South Carolina Nurses
Association
1821 Gadsden Street
Columbia, South
Carolina 29201
(803) 252-4781

Tennessee Nurses
Association
545 Mainstream Drive,
Suite 405
Nashville, Tennessee
37228-1207
(615) 254-0350

Texas Nurses Association
Community Bank Building
300 Highland Mall Boulevard
Suite 300
Austin, Texas 78752-3718
(512) 452-0645

Vermont State
Nurses Association
500 Dorset Street
South Burlington, VT 05403
(802) 864-9390

Virginia Nurses Association
1311 High Point Avenue
Richmond, VA 23230
(804) 353-7311

West Virginia Nurses
Association
1 Players Club Drive,
Building # 3
P.O. Box 1946
Charleston, W V 25327
(304) 342-1169

Utah Nurses Association
1058 A East 900 South
Salt Lake City, Utah
84105
(801) 322-3439

Virgin Islands Nurses
Association
P.O. Box 583
Christiansted
Saint Croix,United States
(809) 773-233 ext. 154

Washington State Nur-
ses Association
2505 Second Avenue,
Suite   500
Seattle, WA 98121
(206) 443-9762

Wisconsin Nurses
Association
6117 Monona Drive
Madison, WI 53716
(608) 221-0383

Wyoming Nurses Association
Majestic Building, Room 305
1603 Capitol Avenue
Cheyenne, WY 82001
(307) 635-3955

Virgin Islands Nurses
Association
P.O. Box 2866
Charlotte Amalie
St.Thomas,Virgin Is-
lands 00801

NURSES ORGANIZATIONS

Aerospace Medical Association
Flight Nurse Section
Washington National Airport
Washington, DC 20001

Alpha Tau Delta
National Fraternity for
Professional Nurses
489 Serento Circle
Thousand Oaks,CA
91360

American Association
of Colleges of Nursing
Suite 430
11 DuPont Circle
Washington, DC 20036

American Association of
Critical Care Nurses
One Civic Plaza
New Port Beach,CA
92660

American Association
of Nephrology Nurses
Box 56
N Woodbury Road
Pitman, NJ 08071

American Association of
Neurological/Neurosurgi-
cal Nurses
Suite 1519
625 N. Michigan Avenue
Chicago, IL 60611

American Association
of Nurse Anesthetists
Suite 929
111 E. Wacker Drive
Chicago, IL 60601

American College
of Nurse Midwives
Suite 1120
1522 K Street NW
Washington, DC 20005

American Holistic
Nurses Association
P.O. Box 116
Telluride, CO 81435

American Indian
Nurses Association
P.O. Box 1588
Norman, OK 73071

American Nurses
Association, Inc.
1101 N. 14th Street, N.W.
Suite 700
Washington, DC 20005

American Society for
Nursing
Service Administrators
840 N Lakeshore Drive
Chicago, IL 60611

Association for Practitioners
in Infection Control
23341 N. Milwaukee Avenue
Half Day, IL 60069

Association of Operat-
ing Room Nurses
10170 E. Mississippi
Avenue
Denver, CO 80231

Association of Pediatric
Oncology Nurses
P.O. Box 7999
San Francisco, CA 94120

Association of
Rehabilitation Nurses
Suite 470
1701 Lake Avenue
Glenview, IL 60025

National Organization for
the Advancement of Associate
Degree Nursing (NOAADN)
Amarillo CollegeP.O. Box 447
Amarillo, TX 79178

Emergency Department
Nurses Association
Suite 1131
666 N. Lakeshore Drive
Chicago, IL 60611

International Association
for Enterostomal Therapy
1701 Lake Avenue
Glenview, IL 60025

InternationalCouncil of
Nurses
3, rue Ancien-Port 1201
Geneva, Switzerland

North American Nursing
Diagnosis Association
Saint Louis University
Department of Nursing
3525 Caroline Street
Saint Louis, MO 63104

North Association of
Hispanic Nurses
4359 S. Rockdale
San Antonio, TX 78233

National Association of
Pediatric Nurses
Associates/Practitioners
Box 56
N. Woodbury Road
Pitman, NJ 08071

National Black Nurses
Association
425 Ohio Building
175 South Main Street
Akron, OH 44308

National Center for
Nursing Ethics
P.O. Box 2237
Cincinnati, OH 45201

National League for
Nursing
10 Columbus Circle
New York,NY 10019

National Male Nurses
Association
2308 State Street
Saginaw, MI 48502

National Nurses
Societyon
 Alcoholism
P.O. Box 7728
Indian Branch Creek
Shawnee Mission, KS
66207

National Student Nurses
 Association
Suite 1325
555 E. 57th Street
New York, NY 10019

Nurses Christian Fellow-
ship
233 Langdon Street
Madison, WI 53703

Oncology Nursing Society
701 Washington Road
Pittsburgh, PA 15228

Orthopedic Nurses Association
Suite 501
1938 Peach Tree Road NW
Atlanta, GA 30309

Sigma Theta Tau
National Honor
Society of Nursing
P.O. Box 1926
Indianapolis, IN
46206-1926

World Health
 Organization
Avenue Appia 1211
Geneva 27, Switzerland

National Licensed Practical
Nurses Educational Foundation
888 7th Avenue
New York, NY 10019

RESOURCES FOR MATERNAL
CARE NURSES

AIDS

AIDS MEDICAL FOUNDATION
10 EAST 13TH Street
Suite LD
New York, NY   10003

BREAST-FEEDING

LaLeche International, Inc.
9616 Minneapolis Avenue
Franklin Park, IL 60123

CHILDBIRTH INFORMATION

American Academy of
Husband-Coached Childbirth
P.O. Box 5224
Sherman Oaks, CA 91413

American College of Home Obstetrics
P.O. Box 25
River Forest, IL 60305

American Society of Childbirth Educators
P.O. Box 16159
7113 Lynwood Drive
Tampa, Florida 33687

American Society for
Psychoprophylaxis in Obstetrics
West 96th Street
New York, NY 10025

Caesarean/Support, Education, and Concern
23 Cedar Street
Cambridge, MA 02140

Childbirth Education Foundation
P.O. Box 37
Appalachin, NY 13732

Childbirth Without Pain
Education Association
20134 Snowden
Detroit, MI 48235

Informed Homebirth
P.O. Box 788
Boulder, CO 80306

Maternity Center Association, Inc.
48 East 92nd Street
New York, New York 10028

FAMILY PLANNING

Planned Parenthood
1220 19th Street, NW
Washington, DC 20036

Zero Population Growth
1346 Connecticut Avenue, NW
Washington, DC 20036

FERTILITY STUDIES

American Fertility Foundation
1608 13th Avenue, S, Suite 101
Birmingham, AL 35205

Fertility Research Foundation
1430 Second Avenue, Suite 103
New York, NY 10021

Surrogate Parenting Associates, Inc.
Suite 222, Doctor's Office Building
250 E. Liberty Street
Louisville, KY 40205

Eastern Virginia Medical School
Norfolk General Hospital

The Howard and Georgeanna Jones
Institute for Reproductive Medicine
304 Medical Tower
Norfolk, VA 23507

GENETIC COUNSELING

National Genetics Foundation
555 W 57th Street
New York, New York 10019

PARENTING AND CONCERNS

American Association for
Marriage and Family Therapy
1717 K St, NW
Suite 407
Washington, DC 20006

Association of Planned Parenthood Professionals
810 Seventh Avenue
New York, NY 10019

Department of Health, Education, and Welfare

US Children's Bureau
Office of Child Development
P.O. Box 1182
Washington, DC 20013

Grief Institute
P.O. Box 623
Englewood, CO 80151

National Center for the Prevention and
Treatment of Child Abuse and Neglect
Department of Pediatrics
University of Colorado Medical Center
1205 Oneida Street
Denver, CO 80220
(National Child Protection Newsletter)

National Committee for Prevention of
Child Abuse
Suite 510
111 East Wacker Drive
Chicago, IL 60601

National Foundation for Sudden Infant Death, Inc.
1501 Broadway
New York, NY 10036

Parenting Materials Information Center
Southwest Educational Development Laboratory
211 E 7th St
Austin, Texas 78701

Parents Anonymous
2810 Artesia Blvd
Redondo Beach, CA 90278

Parents of Premature and High Risk Infants
International
33 W 42nd St, Suite 1227
New York, NY 10036

Parents Without Partners
7910 Woodmont Avenue
Washington, DC 20014

Single Mothers by Choice
501 12th Street
Brooklyn, NY 11215

PROFESSIONAL ORGANIZATIONS

American Association for Maternal and Child
Health
233 Prospect, P-209
La Jolla, CA 92037

American College of Nurse-Midwives
1522 K St, NW
Suite 1120
Washington, DC 20005

American College of Obstetricians
and Gynecologists
600 Maryland Avenue, SW
Suite 300
Washington, DC 20024

American Foundation for Maternal and Child
Health
30 Beekman Place
New York, NY 10022

Maternity Center Association
48 E 92nd Street
New York, NY 10028

PUBLIC HEALTH ORGANIZATIONS

American Public Health Association
1015 15th Street, NW
Washington, DC 20005

American Red Cross
18th and E Streets, NW
Washington, DC 20006

Centers for Disease Control
Atlanta, GA 30333

Medic Alert Foundation
P.O. Box 1009
Turlock, CA 95380

National Institutes of Health
Bethesda, MD 20014

Project HOPE Health Sciences Education Center
Millwood, Va 22646

SEX EDUCATION

Council for Sex Information and Education
Box   23088
Washington, DC 20024

Sex Information and Education Council of the
United States
80 Fifth Avenue, Suite 801
New York, NY 10011

SEXUAL THERAPY

American Association of Sex Educators,
Counselors and Therapists
11 Dupont Circle, Suite 220
Washington, DC 20036

Center for Marital and Sexual Studies
5199 East Pacific Coast HWY
Long Beach, CA 90804

Masters and Johnson Institute
24 South Kings Highway
St Louis, MO 63108

Loyola Sexual Dysfunction Clinic
Loyola University Hospital
2160 S 1st Avenue
Maywood, IL 60153

Society for Sex Therapy
c/o Barry McCarthy, PhD
Department of Psychology
The American University
Washington, DC 20016

SEXUALLY-TRANSMITTED DISEASES

American Social Health Association
260 Sheridan Road
Palo Alto, CA 94306

Herpes Resource Information
Box 100
Palo Alto, CA 94302
National AIDS Hotline
1-800-342-2437

National VD Hotline
1-800-227-8922

APPENDIX A:
PROFESSIONAL
STANDARDS

Appendix A: Professional Standards

UNIVERSAL NURSING PRACTICE STANDARDS

STANDARD I
Nursing Practice

Comprehensive nursing care for women and newborns focuses on helping individuals, families and communities achieve their optimum health potential. This is best achieved within the framework of the nursing process.

The nurse is responsible for decisions and actions within the domain of nursing practice, which may include:

- ❖ Integration of the nursing process components of assessment, planning, implementation, and evaluation in all areas of nursing practice

- ❖ Individualization and prioritization of nursing care to meet the physical, psychological, spiritual and social needs of patients

- ❖ Collaboration with the individual, family, and other members of the health care team

- ❖ Promotion of a safe and therapeutic environment for both the recipients and providers of nursing care

- ❖ Demonstration and validation of competence in nursing practice

- ❖ Acquisition of specialized knowledge and skills and additional formal education to provide specialized care

- ❖ Provision for complete and accurate documentation of care

The written or computerized patient record is the documented means of communication among all members of the health-care team. It also promotes continuity of care and provides a mechanism for recordings of the patient's history and physical examination as well as the nursing plan of care, including goals, interventions, health education and evaluation of patient and family responses. Additional documentation may include planned follow-up and appropriate referrals. All information contained in the patient record and related to the care of the patient and family is confidential and should be released only according to institutional policy.

Note: To apply this universal standard to a sPecific area of gynecologic, obstetric, or neonatal nursing practice, refer directly to the specialty-specific nursing practice standards section.

STANDARD II
Health Education and Counseling

Health education for the individual, family and community is an integral part of comprehensive nursing care. Such education encourages participation in, and shared responsibility for, health promotion, maintenance, and restoration.

Comprehensive health education includes:

❖ Identification of the needs and abilities of the learner

❖ Collaboration with the patient and other health-care providers in design, content, and follow-up of the educational plan

❖ Provision of accurate and current information

- ❖ Provision of information based on educationally sound principles of teaching and learning
- ❖ Recognition of patient rights, responsibilities, and alternative choices
- ❖ Utilization of available educational resources in the practice environment
- ❖ Utilization of available educational resources to provide health education information to individuals/families in the community
- ❖ Documentation and evaluation of health education including patient response

The nurse participates in and/or coordinates the health education and counseling process. It begins with the initial patient contact or admission to the unit or service and is an ongoing, continuous process.

Note: *To apply this universal standard to a specific area of gynecological, obstetric, or neonatal nursing practice, refer directly to the specialty-specific practice standards section.*

STANDARD III
Policies, Procedures and Protocols

Written policies, procedures and protocols clarify the scope of nursing practice and delineate the qualifications of personnel authorized to provide care to women and newborns within the health-care setting.

The components of policies, procedures and protocols are based on

- ❖ Recognition of the organization's philosophy

❖ Recognition of the unit's philosophy

❖ Coordination with the overall mission of the organization

❖ Assessment of the practice setting and determination of types of services to be provided

❖ Incorporation of a multidisciplinary approach in their development

❖ Identification of specific areas of practice to be addressed

❖ Reflection of current practice, standards and local regulations

❖ Anticipated use as references for health-care providers, orientation of new personnel and students, quality assurance activities, and/or guiding nursing actions in emergency situations

The development of policies, procedures, and protocols should include consideration of staff availability, skill and licensure; the physical plant and equipment; effects on other departments; and fiscal impact. Policies, procedures and protocols should be reviewed and revised at least on an annual basis or more frequently as science/technology changes.

Note: To apply this universal standard to a specific area of gynecologic, obstetric, or neonatal nursing practice, refer directly to the specialty-specific nursing practice standards section.

STANDARD IV
Professional Responsibility and Accountability

Comprehensive nursing care for women and newborns is provided by nurses who are clinically competent and accountable for professional actions and legal responsibilities inherent in the nursing role.

Responsibility and accountability for knowledge and competence in nursing practice for women and newborns include:

- ❖ Awareness of changing practices and professional and ethical issues

- ❖ Knowledge and clinical skills gained through in-service education, professional continuing education, research data, and professional literature

- ❖ Implementation of newly acquired knowledge and skills

- ❖ Collaboration through networking and sharing with other professionals

- ❖ Participation in the development of standards and policies, procedures and protocols

- ❖ Participation with professional committees within the institution

- ❖ Participation in periodic peer and self-evaluations

- ❖ Recognition of certification as one mechanism for the demonstration of special knowledge within the specialty area of practice

Legal accountability extends to:

❖ Nurse practice acts

❖ Parameters of professional practice established by professional organizations

❖ Institutional standards

❖ Legislative changes that affect practice

❖ Policies, procedures, and protocols within the practice environment

STANDARD V
Utilization of Nursing Personnel

Nursing care for women and newborns is conducted in practice settings that have qualified nursing staff in sufficient numbers to meet patient-care needs.

Each practice setting should have sufficient nursing personnel to meet patient-care requirements. Nursing staff who provide direct care to women and newborns should be supervised by registered nurses who are clinically proficient in the specialty area of practice. The patient-care unit or service is managed by a professional nurse who is prepared educationally and clinically to assume a leadership position. In all practice settings, the nurse may practice independently or collaboratively with other health-care team members. It is essential that nurses know both the responsibilities and the limitations of professional nursing practice specific to the practice setting.

Many variables are considered in determining both the number and type of nursing staff needed for a practice setting. Among these variables are those related to the patient, practice, organization, and personnel. Patient-related variables may include:

- ❖ Patient demographics and acuity of patients served
- ❖ Length of stay
- ❖ Educational needs
- ❖ Cultural factors and level of comprehension
- ❖ Communication barriers
- ❖ Discharge or home-care needs

Practice-related variables may include:

- ❖ Difference in educational and experiential levels of nursing staff
- ❖ Nursing philosophy
- ❖ Type of nursing-care delivery system
- ❖ Use of assistive personnel
- ❖ Use of nurses in expanding roles
- ❖ Participation in teaching programs

Organizational variables may include

- ❖ Scope of services provided
- ❖ Availability of support services
- ❖ Patient volume
- ❖ Mission or philosophy of organization
- ❖ Risk-management concerns
- ❖ Quality assurance programs
- ❖ Policies, procedures, and protocols
- ❖ Physical plant

- ❖ Marketing strategies and
- ❖ Fiscal considerations

Personnel variables relate to the type and number of professional and nonprofessional staff and may include

- ❖ Education, skill and experience of nursing leadership

Educational preparation, skill and experience of staff

- ❖ Types and mix of nursing staff
- ❖ Availability of qualified alternative staff to deal with emergencies or unanticipated volumes
- ❖ Distribution of staff, e.g. temporary reassignment, floating, on-call, cross training and supplemental staffing
- ❖ Responsibilities for orientation, precepting or students
- ❖ Turnover rates
- ❖ Clerical and technical support

Competency based job descriptions should be available for each level of nursing staff. Orientation for all personnel should include a general overview of organization and specific information about the individual practice setting. Performance evaluations for all personnel should be conducted, documented, and discussed on a regular basis with input from the individual, colleagues and supervisory staff

STANDARD VI
Ethics

Ethical principles guide the process of decision making for nurses caring for women and newborns at all times and especially when personal or professional values conflict with those of the patient, family, colleagues, or practice setting

The nurse should have the opportunity to participate in the ethical decision-making process. To participate actively, nurses should:

- ❖ Clarify their own personal and professional values

- ❖ Recognize the difficulty in selecting a course of action that is morally and ethically acceptable to all parties

- ❖ Communication openly and assertively

- ❖ Identify options

- ❖ Seek consultations

Nurses must carefully examine their own value systems since values influence the decision-making process. Opportunities should be provided in the practice setting for discussion of potential ethical issues. Each practice setting should have a framework for decision making regarding bioethical dilemmas. Ethical dilemmas generally arise when there is a conflict between loyalties, rights, duties or values.

For nurses, most ethical dilemmas occur when there is a real or perceived requirement to act in a manner contrary to personal values or when care ordered or provided does not seem compatible with the best interest of the patient. Common areas of concern may include:

- ❖ Nursing autonomy and decision making

- ❖ Maternal interests versus fetal interests

❖ Issues of duty, obligation and loyalty (for example, employer to employee, professional to public, professional to professional)

❖ Patient's rights to resources, privacy, confidentiality, information, participation in decision making, and refusal of therapy

❖ The right to live or die

❖ Life cycle concerns, including contraception, sterilization, pregnancy termination, genetic manipulation, infanticide, sexuality and choices of life-style, and euthanasia

❖ Fetal or neonatal conditions incompatible with life

❖ Fetal tissue use

❖ Biomedical intervention

The bioethics literature can provide nurses with strategies to cope with or resolve decisions in situations when conflicts of values occur. For ethical decision-making frameworks to be applied to practice situations, working relationships must be established in which individuals may express their own points of view. All persons potentially affected by an ethical decision have the right to participate in the decision-making process.

STANDARD VII
Research

Nurses caring for women and newborns utilize research findings, conduct nursing research, and evaluate nursing practice to improve the outcomes of care

- ❖ Knowledge of the research process and participation in scientific inquiry are necessary to

- ❖ Conduct or participate in the conduct of research according to ethical guidelines

- ❖ Use research findings to provide appropriate and safe nursing care

- ❖ Use research findings as a basis for validating standards of nursing care

- ❖ Evaluate the relevance and application of research findings from nursing and related disciplines

- ❖ Validate the effect of nursing practice of patient outcomes

STANDARD VIIII
Quality Assurance

Quality and appropriateness of patient care are evaluated through a planned assessment program using specific, identified clinical indicators.

Each unit or service should have a written quality assurance plan that reflects a philosophy that is coordinated with the organization's mission and overall quality assurance program. Objectives of the unit-based or service-based quality assurance plan should include:

- ❖ Assurance of consistent quality patient outcomes

- ❖ Identification and correction of potential nursing practice deficiencies

- ❖ Promotion of professional nursing practice based on appropriate nursing standards

❖ Education and participation of staff in quality assurance activities

The unit nurse manager is responsible for developing and implementing the unit-based quality assurance plan. The plan should include:

❖ Responsibilities of all personnel in the quality assurance process

❖ The scope of service provided

❖ Important aspects of care or service involving high-risk, high-volume and problem-prone patients or activities

❖ Clinical indicators or measurable standards that affect the aspects of care and service that have been identified as important

❖ Specific criteria and thresholds for use in monitoring clinical indicators

❖ Methods for the collection and analysis of data, including reference to collection tools, sample size, time frame, and staff responsibility

❖ Determination of appropriate corrective action, when indicated, that will fall into one of three categories: educational, organizational, behavioral change

❖ Follow-up assessment of identified problems

❖ Documentation of all aspects of quality assurance program, including results

❖ A process for communication related to quality assurance activities within the total organization

NEONATAL

STANDARD I
Nursing Practice

Comprehensive neonatal nursing care focuses on helping newborns, families, and communities achieve their optimum health potential. This is best achieved within the framework of the nursing process.

LOW RISK/HEALTHY NEWBORN NURSING PRACTICE

The focus of neonatal nursing is the promotion of maximum health potential for the newborn and family. Nursing care is directed towards anticipating newborns' and families' risk, supporting the neonate through transition to extrauterine life, and facilitating integration of the newborn into the family unit. Nursing interventions address maintenance of expected newborn transition, alterations in the physiological functions of the newborn, and facilitation of newborn/family relationships. Promotion of family integration begins at the first visit during pregnancy and continues throughout the hospital course through home care of the newborn.

Transitional-care practices include a complete history and assessment. Initial assessment and intervention occur concurrently following delivery and may include:

- ❖ Apgar scoring

- ❖ Provision and maintenance of a neutral thermal environment

❖ Establishment and maintenance of cardiopulmonary function

❖ Identification of the at-risk newborn

❖ Identification procedures, including the newborn's legal name

❖ Care of eyes and cord (in accordance with local and institutional regulations) and Vitamin K administration

❖ Physical assessment

❖ Vital signs, including temperature, heart rate, respiratory rate and blood pressure

❖ Gestational age assessment

❖ Routine laboratory assessment

❖ Facilitation of family involvement

❖ Initiation/facilitation of feeding

❖ Infection control using universal precautions

After initial stabilization of the newborn, the neonatal nurse performs an ongoing assessment to provide data for planning the newborn's care. Nursing care follows written policies, procedures and protocols. These are developed by the nursing department, in conjunction with the department of pediatrics and obstetrics, and reflect awareness of professional standards of care. In accordance with these policies, procedures and protocols, the nurse may

❖ Provide nursing interventions to meet the newborn's needs

❖ Review the maternal-fetal and newborn history

❖ Maintain a neutral thermal environment

❖ Perform vital signs, including temperature, heart rate, respiratory rate, and blood pressure

❖ Perform and interpret indicated diagnostic tests

❖ Implement emergency measures, including resuscitation

❖ Collect laboratory specimens as indicated/appropriate

❖ Assist with diagnostic and special procedures

❖ Assume responsibility for medication administration and monitoring

❖ Coordinate, facilitate, and evaluate nutritional status and feeding patterns

❖ Assess the physical, neurological, behavioral, and developmental status of the newborn

❖ Provide the initial bath

❖ Assess behavioral and developmental patterns and care-taking capabilities and abilities of the family unit

❖ Provide the opportunity for the newborn's integration into the family unit

❖ Collaborate with the postpartum nursing staff

❖ Guide referrals for follow-up, including support groups and special home-care needs

With additional formal education and acquisition of specialized knowledge and skill, the professional nurse can assume an expanded role as nurse practitioner. Nurses in expanded practice roles may provide comprehensive health care within the scope of practice as defined by the institution/practice setting and nurse practice acts.

HIGH RISK NEWBORN NURSING PRACTICE

Intensive neonatal nursing care is provided for newborns whose health care needs cannot be met in the healthy/low risk newborn unit. Nursing care of the newborn begins with anticipation and identification of high-risk newborns. The focus of neonatal nursing is the promotion of maximum health potential for the neonate and family

Nursing interventions address alterations in the physiologic functions of the newborn and alterations in family processes. Promotion of family integration begins during pregnancy and continues throughout the hospital course and through home care of the newborn.

The initial assessment and interventions for the high-risk newborn may include:

- ◆ Apgar scoring
- ◆ Provision and maintenance of a neutral, thermal environment
- ◆ Establishment and maintenance of cardiopulmonary function
- ◆ Identification procedures
- ◆ Care of eyes and cord (in accordance with local and institutional regulations) and Vitamin K administration
- ◆ Physical assessment, including weight and length

* Vital signs including temperature, heart rate, respiratory rate, and blood pressure
* Gestational age assessment
* Routine and indicated laboratory tests
* Establishment of parenteral therapy
* Provision and maintenance of fluid and electrolyte balance
* Review of pertinent maternal history
* Infection control using universal precautions
* Preparation for transport if necessary, which includes obtaining parental consent, initiating contact with the transport team and receiving facility, duplicating newborn and maternal records, obtaining cord blood samples and placenta (if appropriate), and facilitating family contact
* Facilitating family involvement
* After initial assessment and stabilization of the high-risk newborn, the nurse performs ongoing assessments to provide data for a nursing diagnosis and to serve as a basis for planning the newborn's care. This plan of care should be reviewed periodically and revised as necessary. Ongoing nursing assessments may include
* Immediate physical needs
* The physical, neurological, behavioral and developmental status of the neonate
* Emotional and developmental status of the family

❖ Family-newborn interaction

❖ The family's understanding of, and response to, the neonate's condition

❖ Socioeconomic and cultural factors

The nurse performs ongoing interventions that may include:

❖ Assisting the family in coping with the newborn's condition

❖ Assisting with technical procedures as delineated by policies, procedures and protocols

❖ Administering fluids and electrolytes, including blood and blood products

❖ Administering medications with awareness of potential side effects

❖ Setting up, calibrating, and applying biomedical equipment and evaluating data

❖ Utilizing laboratory, radiologic, ultrasound, and other diagnostic data in providing care

❖ Initiating and maintaining oxygen/respiratory therapy

❖ Monitoring physical, neurological, behavioral, and developmental status

❖ Obtaining central or peripheral blood samples for cultures, gases, and other lab analyses

❖ Participating in complex care

❖ Performing endotracheal suctioning

❖ Performing chest physiotherapy

- ❖ Performing peripheral venipuncture for administration of fluids or obtaining blood specimens
- ❖ Performing urethral catheterization
- ❖ Monitoring nutritional status and providing nutrition
- ❖ Providing and maintaining a protective environment
- ❖ Managing pain
- ❖ Monitoring and maintaining the neutral thermal environment
- ❖ Implementing emergency procedures
- ❖ Maintaining infection control measures, including hand washing and universal precautions
- ❖ Providing the opportunity for the newborn's integration into the family unit
- ❖ Initiating and participating in neonatal-care conferences with the family and other members of the health-care team
- ❖ Developing and evaluating discharge plans with appropriate referrals
- ❖ Participating in transport services

With additional formal education and the acquisition of specialized knowledge and skill, the professional nurse can assume an expanded role as a nurse practitioner. Nurses in expanded practice roles may provide comprehensive health care within the scope of practice as defined by the institution/practice setting and nurse practice acts.

DISCHARGE/HOME CARE NURSING PRACTICE OF THE LOW AND HIGH RISK NEWBORN

The nurse may coordinate and/or participate in the care of the newborn and family at one or more points in the health-care continuum from illness to follow-up care in the home. Discharge planning and home care should ensure safety of the mother and infant and promote functioning of the family unit. Discharge planning, which should begin on admission, focuses on infant readiness, parent/caretaker and family readiness, and environmental adequacy. The elements of discharge planning are:

1. Infant readiness

❖ Demonstrates physiological stability appropriate to the newborn's condition

2. Parent/caretaker and family readiness

❖ Demonstrates ability and/or knowledge of newborn care including

❖ Bathing

❖ Hair and scalp care

❖ Elimination patterns

❖ Skin and nail care

❖ Eye care

❖ Cord care

❖ Infant sleeping patterns

❖ Vitamin supplement

❖ Feeding and formula preparation

❖ Plans for follow-up medical care

❖ Genitalia and circumcision care

- ❖ Handling of the newborn
- ❖ Growth and development
- ❖ Reactions of siblings
- ❖ Signs and symptoms of illness and when to call the healthcare provider
- ❖ Demonstrates knowledge of specialized care appropriate to the newborn's condition that may include:
- ❖ Phototherapy
- ❖ Oxygen therapy
- ❖ Medication administration
- ❖ Wound care
- ❖ Cardiopulmonaryresuscitation
- ❖ Home respiratory care or monitoring
- ❖ Demonstrates knowledge of preventive care, including:

- · Car seat use
- · Temperature taking in the newborn
- · Home safety

- · Immunizations
- · Signs and symptoms of illness

3. Environmental adequacy

- ❖ Basic facilities for providing newborn care
- ❖ Safety
- ❖ Specialized equipment required for the infant in the home

Post-discharge, a review of significant past history prior to conducting home or follow-up visit is essential. Home care focuses on infant wellness, parent/caretaker and family wellness, and environmental adequacy. A review of pertinent newborn history prior to the follow-up visit may include:

- ❖ Apgar score and delivery history
- ❖ Date of birth and birth weight
- ❖ Serum glucose level, hematocrit, and blood type (if applicable)
- ❖ Date and time of metabolic screen (second screen may be necessary)
- ❖ Demographic information including name, address, telephone number and family location at time of visit
- ❖ Feeding patterns
- ❖ Gestational age
- ❖ Information on cord care and circumcision (if applicable)
- ❖ Family dynamics, home support systems, sibling status, financial status
- ❖ Sleep/wake patterns
- ❖ Significant physical exam findings
- ❖ Weight, length and head circumference measurements and percentiles at discharge

Aspects evaluated in the home visit may include:

1. Infant well being

- ❖ Physical well-being, including physical examination and weight gain
- ❖ Developmental and behavioral status
- ❖ Nutritional status, feeding and elimination patterns
- ❖ Potential for complications
- ❖ Special needs being met

2. Parent/caretaker and family well being:

- ❖ Caretaking abilities, including infant receiving follow-up care
- ❖ Coping and adaptation skills, including: parent/infant interaction, including normal characteristics and barriers
- ❖ Parent responses to stress and crisis
- ❖ Sibling response and intervention
- ❖ Decision-making process
- ❖ Financial resources
- ❖ Support systems, including
- ❖ Integration of infant into family unit
- ❖ Role of extended family
- ❖ Use of community resources, including emergency facilities

3. Environmental adequacy

- ❖ Basic facilities (for example, heat, running water, etc.)
- ❖ Special equipment required by the infant
- ❖ Access to telephone communication
- ❖ Safety

With additional formal education and the acquisition of specialized knowledge and skill, the professional nurse can assume an expanded role as a nurse practitioner. Nurses in expanded practice roles may provide comprehensive health care within the scope of practice as defined by the institution/practice setting and nurse practice acts.

STANDARD II
Health Education and Counseling

Health education for the newborn, family and community is an integral part of comprehensive nursing care. It encourages participation and shared responsibility for health promotion, maintenance and restoration.

LOW-RISK/HEALTHY NEWBORN AND HIGH-RISK NEWBORN HEALTH EDUCATION AND COUNSELING

Health education and counseling for the childbearing and childrearing family may include:

- ❖ Pathophysiological processes
- ❖ Relinquishment
- ❖ Perinatal loss
- ❖ Adolescent parenting

❖ Family dynamics, such as single parenting, siblings and newborns and extended families

❖ Health promotion and maintenance, including growth and development and immunizations

❖ Infant responses and interactions with others

❖ Medication administration

❖ Need for follow-up care and identification of hospital, community and other resources

❖ Feeding practices or choices

❖ Newborn care such as:

· Bathing	· Skin care
· Cord care	· Nail care
· Dressing	· Diapering
· Elimination	· Care of genitalia
· Diaper rash	· Use of thermometer
· Use of bulb syringe	· Positioning

❖ Signs of illness, including jaundice

❖ Newborn nutrition and feeding practices such as:

❖ Breastfeeding, including breastfeeding routines, positioning, sore nipples, fussy newborns, engorgement, plugged ducts, and mastitis, supplements, pumping and storage, signs that breastfeeding is going well, and when to introduce solid foods

❖ Bottlefeeding, including positioning, frequency and amount, mixing formulas, cleaning bottles, introduction of solid foods, fussy newborns, and breast care

❖ Newborn safety, environmental and emergency measures, which may include choking and cardiopulmonary resuscitation, carseat use, pets, and other home environmental issues

DISCHARGE/HOME CARE HEALTH EDUCATION AND COUNSELING FOR THE LOW- AND HIGH-RISK NEWBORN

Health education and counseling in preparation for discharge or for home care of the newborn may include:

❖ Newborn care

❖ Newborn nutrition and feeding practices

❖ Newborn protection and safety

❖ Parenting skills

❖ Infant responses and interactions with others

❖ Family dynamics

❖ Hospital, community and other resources

❖ Pediatric health promotion and maintenance

❖ Newborn growth and development

❖ Immunizations

❖ Use and maintenance of necessary equipment

STANDARD III
POLICIES, PROCEDURES AND PROTOCOLS

Written policies, procedures, and protocols clarify the scope of nursing practice and delineate the qualifications of personnel authorized to provide care to the newborn within the health-care setting

LOW-RISK/HEALTHY NEWBORN POLICIES, PROCEDURES AND PROTOCOLS

Policies, procedures and protocols for the low-risk/healthy newborn nursery may include:

- ❖ Admission criteria
- ❖ Physical assessment parameters
- ❖ Transitional care
- ❖ Routine care, including eye and cord care (in accordance with local and institutional regulations) and Vitamin K administration
- ❖ Vital signs
- ❖ Length, weight, and head circumference
- ❖ Identification of the newborn
- ❖ Indication for, and initiation of, diagnostic assessments
- ❖ Newborn nutrition
- ❖ Medication administration
- ❖ Circumcision, including assistance with procedure and follow-up care
- ❖ Bathing
- ❖ Heelstick for capillary blood assessment

- ❖ Venipuncture for obtaining blood specimens
- ❖ Oral/nasal suctioning
- ❖ Phototherapy
- ❖ Management of intravenous lines
- ❖ Metabolic screening, including genetic screening
- ❖ Use of pulse oximetry
- ❖ Care of physiologic alterations in the newborn, including:

  - Drug/substance withdrawal
  - Congenitalhipdysplasia
  - Circumcision complications
  - Hypoglycemia
  - Polycythemia
  - Feeding intolerance
  - Unusual physical findings
  - (extra digits, skin tags, hemangiomas)

  - Cardiac murmurs
  - Respiratory distress
  - Alterations in skin integrity
  - Hypothermia
  - Anemia
  - Congenital anomalies

- ❖ Screening tests, including hearing
- ❖ Preparation for transport
- ❖ Scope of practice of health-care providers
- ❖ Organizational structure of unit
- ❖ Functional responsibilities of nursing, medical and ancillary personnel
- ❖ Nursing orders and institutional standards of care
- ❖ Patient admission, transfer, discharge and readmission

- Rooming-in
- Nurse's role in research
- Infection surveillance, hand washing, universal precautions, isolation and traffic control
- Visitation
- Setting up, calibrating, and trouble shooting biomedical equipment
- Documentation and record-keeping requirements
- Lines of authority and responsibility (chain of command)
- Hazardous materials
- Relinquishment
- Identification of parenting problems
- Identification of consultation and referral resources and the referral process
- Use and maintenance of department equipment and supplies

Management of neonatal complications and emergencies must be identified in written department policies, procedures, and protocols and may include:

- Cardiopulmonary distress and arrest
- Central nervous system alterations
- Drug/substance withdrawal
- Metabolic alterations
- Respiratory/oxygen therapy initiation
- Thermal alterations

❖ Transfer to an intensive care unit

❖ X-ray, ultrasound and other diagnostic testing

HIGH-RISK NEWBORN POLICIES, PROCEDURES, AND PROTOCOLS

Policies, procedures and protocols for the high-risk or neonatal intensive care unit may include:

❖ Admission assessment

❖ Administration of blood and blood products

❖ Vital signs and hemodynamic monitoring assessments

❖ Measurement of length, weight and abdominal and head circumference

❖ Administration of medications and parenteral therapy

❖ Administration of oxygen and respiratory therapy

❖ Assistance with technical procedures

❖ Cardiopulmonary distress and arrest

❖ Care of central arterial and venous lines

❖ Care of chest tubes

❖ Endotracheal intubation and care of intubated infants

❖ Assisting with eye examinations

❖ Hearing screening

❖ Hyperalimentation

- ❖ Setting up, applying and trouble shooting biomedical equipment
- ❖ Infant demise
- ❖ Assisting with insertion and care of peripheral and central lines
- ❖ Maintenance of tracheostomy tubes
- ❖ Metabolic alterations
- ❖ Care of physiologic alterations in the newborn, including
- ❖ Craniosynostosis
- ❖ Intraventricular hemorrhage
- ❖ Periventricular leukomalacia
- ❖ Seizures
- ❖ Anomalies and syndromes
- ❖ Congenital heart disease
- ❖ Drug/substance withdrawal
- ❖ Respiratory problems, including persistent pulmonary hypertension, diaphragmatic hernia, hyaline membrane disease, bronchopulmonary dysplasia, pulmonary air leaks, meconium aspiration, and pneumonia
- ❖ Necrotizing enterocolitis
- ❖ Acute renal failure/acute tubular necrosis
- ❖ Esophagal atresia with or without tracheal esophageal fistulae

- Metabolic problems such as hypoglycemia, hypocalcemia, and hyperbilirubinemia
- Hematologic problems such as isoimmunization, anemia, and disseminated intravascular coagulation
- Hypothermia/hyperthermia
- Retinopathy of prematurity
- Phototherapy
- Pulse oximetry
- Perioperative care
- Bathing
- Suctioning/chest physiotherapy procedures
- Ostomy care
- Thermoregulation
- Immunization
- Admission, transfer, discharge and readmission of patients
- Designation of responsible individuals for attendance at deliveries and resuscitation teams
- Documentation and record-keeping requirements
- Organizational structure of the unit
- Infection surveillance, hand washing, isolation, universal precautions, and traffic control
- Hazardous materials
- Nurse's role in research
- Nurse's role regarding patient consent

- ❖ Nursing orders and standards of care
- ❖ Scope of practice of health care providers
- ❖ Transport procedures, including roles and responsibilities of the transport team
- ❖ Use and maintenance of department equipment and supplies
- ❖ Discharge planning and home care
- ❖ Identification of consultations, referrals, resources, and processes
- ❖ Identification procedures for the newborn
- ❖ Parent health education
- ❖ Perinatal loss
- ❖ Spiritual care of the family

DISCHARGE/HOME CARE POLICIES, PROCE-DURES AND PROTOCOLS FOR THE LOW- AND HIGH-RISK NEWBORN

The need for ongoing care of the newborn outside the hospital setting may arise as part of the overall perinatal program or because of a specific condition of the newborn for which professional assistance is necessary following discharge. Policies, procedures and protocols may include

- ❖ Assessment of the newborn
- ❖ Management of common problems found at neonatal home visits
- ❖ Eligibility criteria for enrollment in early discharge programs and/or follow-up programs
- ❖ Home apnea monitoring

❖ Home oxygen or respiratory therapy

❖ Home phototherapy

❖ Medication administration

❖ Home-visit standards of care and documentation and

❖ Maternity short-stay program criteria for early discharge less than 24 hours, i.e., uncomplicated prenatal, intrapartum, or postpartum course, stable newborn, family members or support persons available to mother; maternal readiness for self-care; newborn care established; and procedures/criteria for readmission established.

By the *Association of Women's Health, Obstetric and Neonatal Nursing.* These standards are reviewed every five years and revised as necessary.

The following information provides information on specific areas of competency expected of each nurse who uses fetal surveillance techniques in assessing, promoting and evaluating maternal and fetal well being during the antepartum and intrapartum stages of pregnancy. The information presented herein also sets guidelines for educational programs containing a core curriculum of essential principles necessary for minimum competency and ongoing instruction to maintain competency in the area of using fetal monitoring techniques. Additionally, nurses should be familiar with the policies of the institutions where they work or matriculate, and should refer to this policy and nurse practice acts as they pertain to fetal heart monitoring and fetal surveillance.

ANTEPARTUM FETAL SURVEILLANCE

Nursing Practice Competencies

Nurses with responsibility for performing antepartum fetal surveillance should demonstrate competency in the application and use of external electronic and auscultatory fetal monitoring equipment and interpretation of data. Before assuming responsibility for antepartum monitoring, the nurse should be able to:

❖ Describe antepartum testing criteria and indications for testing, for example, high-risk pregnancy

❖ Provide patient education regarding the procedure and its purpose

❖ Prepare the patient, perform complete assessment including Leopold's maneuvers, palpate the fundus, and apply the external electronic fetal monitor

❖ Recognize contraindications to the use of oxytocin and nipple stimulation

❖ Conduct the prescribed antepartum tests

❖ Implement interventions per protocol for nonreassuring findings

❖ Communicate the content of electronic fetal monitoring data for final interpretation in accordance with institutional policy

❖ Document appropriate entries in the written or computerized patient record, and the electronic fetal monitor tracing or storage disk

❖ Discontinue electronic fetal monitoring according to the institutional policy, procedure, and protocol

❖ Communicate appropriate follow-up information to the patient

Biophysical profile components including fetal movement, tone, breathing, and amniotic fluid volume, and other ultrasound assessments such as fetal position and placental grading and location may be performed in accordance with institutional policy and nurse practice act after appropriate educational and clinical instruction in the technique

Educational Guidelines

Three to four hours of didactic instruction specific to antepartum fetal heart monitoring is considered the minimal requirement. Didactic instruction should be followed by supervised clinical experience prior to independent nursing practice. The period of supervised clinical experience required to achieve competency varies with the individual and the practice setting.

Additional didactic instruction and supervised clinical experience specific to antepartum fetal surveillance with ultrasound will vary with the individual and the practice setting.

Didactic Content Outline

I. *Elements of antepartum fetal surveillance*

- Maternal-fetal physiology
- Indications for testing
- Methods and interpretation
- Nonstress test
- Contraction stress tests
- Spontaneous

- Nipple stimulation
- Oxytocin
- Ultrasound evaluation, biophysical profile, and other similar noninvasive assessments according to institutional policy and nurse practice acts
- Contrainidications for use of oxytocin and nipple stimulation

II. *Patient education*

- Indication for testing
- Test procedure
- Test results
- Follow-up

III. *Nurse accountability*

- Policies, procedures and protocols
- Standards of practice
- Follow-up, interpretation and reporting protocol
- Documentation in the written or computerized patient record and on the electronic fetal monitor tracing or storage disk
- Legal and ethical issues
- Lines of authority and responsibility (chain of command)

Clinical Learning Experiences and Evaluation

The sequence and specific nature of clinical learning experience can be adapted to accommodate clinical instructors' or preceptors' styles and individual learners' needs.

Practice sessions should include a policy, procedure and protocol manual review and also may include:

- ❖ Electronic fetal monitor tracing review sessions

- ❖ Small group discussion/case studies
- ❖ Clinical conferences (multidisciplinary)
- ❖ Role-play situations
- ❖ Videotaped observations and follow-up discussion
- ❖ Computer simulation
- ❖ One-to-one tutorial
- ❖ Self-study

Practicum

- ❖ Demonstration with return demonstration of equipment, set-up, application and calibration
- ❖ Demonstration with return demonstration of equipment maintenance

Clinical application of the nursing process under the supervision of the instructor or preceptor:

- ❖ Instruction of the patient and family
- ❖ Selection of the method of assessment
- ❖ Application of technology (including calibration)
- ❖ Recognition of errors and limitations of technology
- ❖ Formulation of a nursing diagnosis or nursing problem
- ❖ Intervention
- ❖ Documentation in the written or computerized patient record and on the electronic fetal monitor tracing or storage disk

❖ Evaluation and follow-up

Competency Validation

Evaluation of didactic and clinical learning validates competency. Evaluation can be ongoing during the learning process or conducted at the conclusion of the learning experiences. The components that comprise competency validation include:

Written or verbal exercises such as:

❖ Examination

❖ Case study analysis

❖ Electronic fetal monitor tracing interpretation sessions

❖ Interpretation of hospital policies, procedures, and protocols

❖ Identification of appropriate lines of authority and responsibility (chain of command)

❖ Observation by instructor or preceptor of nurse providing patient care in fetal heart monitoring clinical situations

❖ Documentation of competency in the fetal surveillance technique before the nurse functions independently.

Intrapartum Fetal Heart Monitoring

Nurse Practice Competencies

To function competently in the use of intrapartum fetal heart monitoring, the nurse should demonstrate competency in the application and use of auscultatory and electronic fetal monitoring equipment and interpretation of data. The intrapartum nurse should therefore be able to:

- ❖ Implement the appropriate fetal heart monitoring method based on patient status, hospital policy and current standards of practice recommended by professional organizations

- ❖ Explain the principles of the chosen method of fetal heart monitoring to the patient and her support persons

- ❖ Identify the limitations of information produced by each method of monitoring

- ❖ Demonstrate competency in fetal heart monitoring by auscultation

Demonstrate use of electronic fetal monitor:

- ❖ Perform complete assessment including Leopold's maneuvers to determine fetal position and palpate the fundus to determine appropriate site for auscultation

- ❖ Apply fetoscope or Doppler device to the appropriate site

- ❖ Palpate uterine contractions for frequency, duration, and intensity; confirm uterine rest between contractions, determine if abnormal findings are present

❖ Identify and determine the baseline fetal heart rate and rhythm

❖ Identify the presence of fetal heart rate changes with or between uterine contractions

❖ Determine if findings are reassuring or nonreassuring and implement appropriate nursing interventions, including additional fetal monitoring methods

❖ Identify the clinical situations, based on fetal heart monitoring findings, in which immediate notification of the primary health-care provider is appopriate

❖ Communicate the findings from auscultation, interpretation of findings, and resulting nursing intervention (s), in written and verbal form in an appropriate and timely manner.

❖ Document appropriate entries on the written or computerized patient record

❖ Demonstrate appropriate maintenance of auscultation equipment

Demonstrate use of electronic fetal monitor:

❖ Perform complete assessment including Leopold's maneuvers, palpate the fundus, and auscultate the fetal heart rate prior to application of the transducers

❖ Apply external transducers and adjust the electronic fetal monitor accordingly

- ❖ Prepare the patient, set up the equipment, and complete connections for fetal electrode with and without intrauterine pressure catheter

- ❖ Calibrate the monitor for the use of the intrauterine pressure catheter

- ❖ Identify technically inadequate tracings and take appropriate corrective action

- ❖ Obtain and maintain an adequate tracing of the fetal heart and uterine contractions

- ❖ Interpret uterine contraction frequency, duration, intensity, and baseline resting tone as appropriate based on monitoring

- ❖ Identify baseline fetal heart rate and rhythm, variability, and the presence of periodic and nonperiodic changes

- ❖ Determine if findings are reassuring or nonreassuring and implement appropriate nursing interventions

- ❖ Identify the clinical situations, based on fetal heart monitoring findings, in which immediate notification of the primary health-care provider is appropriate

- ❖ Communicate the content of electronic fetal monitoring data, interpretation of data, and resulting nursing intervention(s) in written and verbal form, in an appropriate and timely manner

- ❖ Document appropriate entries in the written or computerized patient record, and on the electronic fetal monitoring tracing or storage disk

❖ Demonstrate appropriate maintenance of electronic fetal monitoring equipment

❖ Demonstrate appropriate storage and retrieval of fetal heart monitoring data

Educational Guidelines

The content of educational programs specific to intrapartum fetal heart monitoring should include didactic instruction to meet nursing practice competencies, followed by a period of supervised clinical experience prior to independent nursing practice. The format for presenting didactic instruction may vary depending on content objectives.   A minimum of eight hours is recommended to cover the core instructional content.

The period of supervised clinical experience required to achieve competency may vary with the individual. As with the core content, ongoing instructional programs may be adapted as necessary to accommodate instructors' and individual learners' needs.

Didactic Content Outline

I.   Introduction to fetal heart monitoring

A. Goals of fetal heart monitoring

1. Determine fetal heart rate characteristics and uterine activity

2. Assess fetal well-being

B. Methods of monitoring

1. Auscultation and palpation

2. Electronic fetal monitoring

      a. Continuous
      b. Intermittent
   3. Combination of methods

II. **Elements of instrumentation and assessment**

   A.Uterine activity and monitoring

     1. Palpation
        a. Principles
        b. Techniques
        c. Sources of error and limitations
        d. Benefits and risks
     2. External electronic tocodynamometer
        a. Principles
        b. Application and care during use
        c. Sources of error and limitations
        d. Benefits and risks
     3. Internal electronic intrauterine pressure catheter
        a. Types and principles
           1. Fluid-filled catheters
           2. Transducer-tipped catheters
        b. Application and care during use
        c. Calibration
        d. Sources of error
        e. Benefits and risks

   B.Fetal Heart Rate

     1. External auscultation
        a. Types and principles
           1. Doppler
           2. Fetoscope
        b. Techniques
        c. Sources of error and limitations
        d. Benefits and risks

2. External electronic ultrasound transducer
    a. Principles of Doppler/ultrasound
    b. Application and care during use
    c. Sources of error and limitations
    d. Benefits and risks
3. Internal electronic: fetal electrode
    a. Principles of cardiotachometry
    b. Application/care during use
    c. Sources of error and limitations
    d. Benefits and risks

III. **Fetal oxygenation**
A. Physiology of fetal oxygenation
    1. Uteroplacental circulation
    2. Exchange mechanisms
    3. Effects of uterine contractions
    4. Acid-base homeostasis
B. **Pathophysiology of fetal oxygenation**
    1. Maternal
        a. Impaired circulation
        b. Impaired oxygen exchange
    2. Uterine contractions
        a. Endogenous causes
        b. Exogenous causes
    3. Placental
        a. Impaired circulation
        b. Impaired oxygen exchange
    4. Umbilical cord
        a. Compression
        b. Occlusion
        c. Compromised perfusion

   5. Fetal
      a. Impaired circulation
      b. Impaired oxygen exchange

IV. Interpretation of fetal heart monitoring data

   A. Uterine activity
      1. Resting tone
      2. Contraction frequency
      3. Contraction duration
      4. Contraction intensity
   B. Baseline fetal heart rate and rhythm
      1. Rate and rhythm
         a. Mechanism (intrinsic and extrinsic control)
            1. Nervous system control
            2. Myocardial control
            3. Endocrine control
            4. Gestational age influence
         b. Interpretation
            1. Normal
            2. Abnormal
               a. Tachycardia
               b. Bradycardia
               c. Dysrhythmia/Arrhythmia
               d. Sinusoidal and pseudo-sinusoidal*
      2. Variability*: short- and long-term
         a. Mechanism
         b. Interpretation
            1. Reassuring
            2. Nonreassuring

C. Periodic fetal heart rate changes*
  1. Accelerations
    a. Characteristics
    b. Mechanisms
    c. Significance
  2. Early decelerations
    a. Characteristics
    b. Mechanisms
    c. Significance
  3. Late decelerations
    a. Characteristics
    b. Mechanisms
    c. Significance
  4. Variable decelerations
    a. Characteristics
    b. Mechanisms
    c. Significance
  5. Prolonged decelerations
    a. Characteristics
    b. Mechanisms
    c. Significance

D. Non-periodic fetal heart rate changes*
  1. Accelerations
    a. Characteristics
    b. Mechanisms
    c. Significance

    2. Variable decelerations
        a. Characteristics
        b. Mechanisms
        c. Significance
    3. Prolonged decelerations
        a. Characteristics
        b. Mechanisms
        c. Significance

E. Auscultated fetal heart changes
    1. Numerical rate
    2. Rhythm
    3. Gradual increase or decrease
    4. Abrupt increase or decrease

V. **Nursing process**

  A. Assessment
    a. Review of prenatal history
    b. Clinical status of the mother and fetus
    c. Fetal heart rate characteristics and interpretation
    d. Uterine contraction characteristics and interpretation
    e. Documentation

  B. Diagnosis
    a. Reassuring
    b. Nonreassuring

  C. Planning and intervention
    1. Independent nursing actions
    2 Fetal heart monitoring findings necessitating immediate notification of primary health care provider
    3. Documentation

4. Nursing accountability
   a. Policies, procedures and protocols
   b. Standards of practice
   c. Legal and ethical issues
   d. Lines of authority and responsibility (chain of command)

D. Evaluation
   1. Response to intervention
   2. Documentation
   3. Continuing plan of nursing care based on response to intervention

Clinical Learning Experiences and Evaluation

The suggested clinical learning experiences and evaluation exercises (under "Antepartum Fetal Surveillance") are also appropriate techniques to achieve competency in intrapartum fetal heart monitoring

Competency Validation

The suggested competency validation exercises (under "Antepartum Fetal Surveillance") are also appropriate techniques to validate competency in intrapartum fetal heart monitoring.

These guidelines are for educational preparation to achieve competency in fetal heart monitoring. Nurses should participate annually in reviews and clinical update sessions to maintain competency in fetal heart monitoring and should take part in the clinical learning experiences. Maintaining the quality of individual practice in accordance with current guidelines and standards is an inherent responsibility of the professional nurse.

AMERICAN NURSES' ASSOCIATION STANDARDS OF MATERNAL AND CHILD HEALTH NURSING PRACTICE

Standard I

The nurse helps children and parents attain and maintain optimum health.

Standard II

The nurse assists families to achieve and maintain optimum health.

Standard III

The nurse assists families to achieve and maintain a balance between the personal growth needs of individual family members and optimum family functioning.

Standard IV

The nurse intervenes with vulnerable clients and families at risk to prevent potential developmental and health problems.

Standard V

The nurse promotes an environment free of hazards to reproduction, growth and development, wellness, and recovery from illness.

Standard VI

The nurse detects changes in health status and deviations from optimum development.

Standard VII

The nurse carries out appropriate interventions and treatment to facilitate survival and recovery from illness.

Standard VIII

The nurse assists clients and families to understand and cope with developmental and traumatic situations during illness, childbearing, childrearing, and childhood.

StandardIX

The nurse actively pursues strategies to enhance access to and utilization of adequate healthcare services.

Standard X

The nurse improves maternal and child health nursing practice through evaluation of practice, education, and research.

Association of Women's Health, Obstetric and Neonatal Nursing

APPENDIX B:
CERVICAL
DILATATION

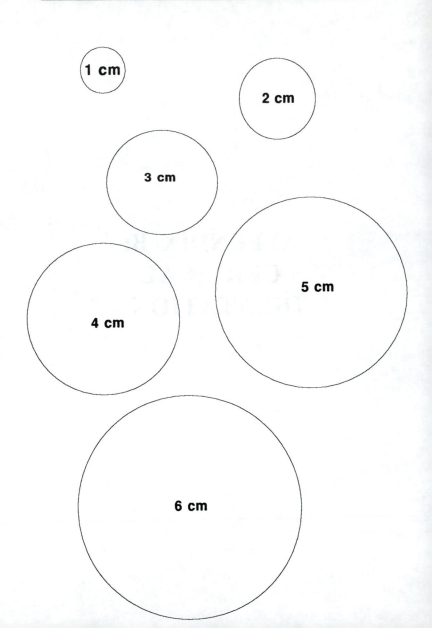

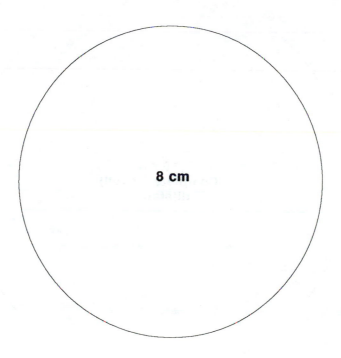

8 cm

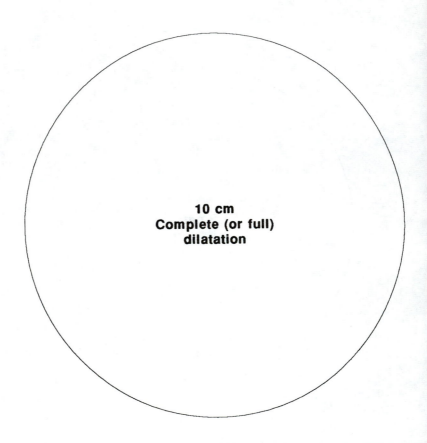

**10 cm
Complete (or full)
dilatation**

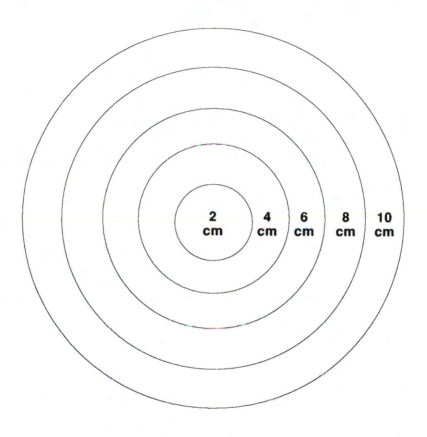

INDEX

V

W

Y

Z

Skidmore-Roth Publishing, Inc. Order Form
1(800) 825-3150

Qty.	Title	Price	Total
	1994 Nurse's Trivia Calendar	$9.95	
	RN NCLEX Review Cards, 2nd Ed.	$24.95	
	PN/VN Review Cards	$24.95	
	Nurse's Survival Guide, 2nd Ed.	$24.95	
	The Body in Brief, 2nd Ed.	$26.95	
	The OSHA Handbook	$79.95	
	The OBRA Guidelines for Quality Improvement in Long Term Care	59.95	
	Diagnostic & Laboratory Cards, 2nd Ed.	$23.95	
	Drug Comparison Handbook	$29.95	
Tax of 8.25% applies to Texas residentsonly. UPS ground shipping $5 for first item, $1 each additional item.		Subtotal	
(Continued on back)		8.25% Tax	
		Shipping	
		TOTAL	

Name
Company
Address
City
State   Zip
Phone
_____ Check enclosed_____ Visa_____ MasterCard
Credit Card Number
Card Holder Name
Signature   Expiration Date

For fastest service call, 1-800-825-3150 or fax your order to us at (915) 877-4424. Orders are accepted by mail.   Prices subject to change without notice.

Skidmore-Roth Publishing, Inc.
7730 Trade Center Avenue
El Paso, TX 79912